FRONTIERS

IN

COMPARATIVE

MEDICINE

W. I. B. BEVERIDGE, D.V.Sc.

Foreword by
ROBERT A. GOOD, M.D., Ph.D.

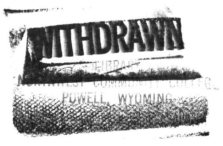
UNIVERSITY OF MINNESOTA PRESS
Minneapolis

Library of Congress Catalog Card Number: 72-79500
ISBN 0-8166-0643-9

Frontiers in Comparative Medicine

THE
WESLEY W. SPINK
LECTURES ON
COMPARATIVE MEDICINE
Volume I

CONTENTS

The Wesley W. Spink Lectures on Comparative Medicine, established in honor of Dr. Spink's wide range of accomplishments, are presented by international authorities in comparative medicine and biology. Sponsorship of the lectures jointly by Carleton College and the University of Minnesota reflects the concern of both institutions for the dissemination of scientific knowledge. The lectures, and the publication of the volumes based on them, have been assisted by grants from the Bush Foundation and Eli Lilly and Company.

FOREWORD

For more than a third of a century at the University of Minnesota, Wesley W. Spink—clinician, internist concerned with the broad realm of infectious disease in man, and experimental pathologist—has been directing his major energies to research on brucellosis. Driven certainly by the Oslerian concept "Know one disease completely and you know all of medicine," Dr. Spink has contributed to the methods of diagnosis, the analysis of the pathogenetic mechanism, and the means of treatment and prevention of brucellosis. To achieve these goals, in different stages of inquiry he has had to be an anatomist, physiologist, pathologist, experimental pathologist, microbiologist, epidemiologist, immunobiologist, diagnostician, compassionate therapist, and practical developer of vaccines—and sometimes all of them at once.

His inquiry has led to questions such as these: What is unique and what is common as this disease is expressed in cattle, goats, sheep, horses, dogs, or humans? What are the manifestations and mechanisms of disease in each species?

Why and when do granulomas form in the organs of domestic and experimental animals and in man? How do hypersensitivity and immunity relate to expressions of disease in acute and chronic illness?

Exploring the many questions derived from his constant efforts to compare human and animal disease has led Dr. Spink to numerous fundamental insights. Some of his many contributions are related to the basis for continuing bacterial infection, the role of endotoxins in symptom and lesion formation, the pathologic physiology of shock, the special significance of IgG antibody levels in diagnosis of ongoing infection, and the role delayed allergy plays in the development of granulomas, rashes, and febrile responses.

No discipline has been too difficult for Dr. Spink to master. No species has been too mundane to study if comparison promised information new and useful to the understanding of brucellosis. Thus, it is entirely fitting that the Wesley W. Spink Lectures should be planned to focus on comparative medicine. Biennially the Spink Lectures will bring to Minnesota one of the world's leading scholars to deliver a series of lectures on this subject that by its very nature transcends artificial boundaries between disciplines which sometimes act as impediments to progress.

The Spink Lectures cut across artificial boundaries of another kind. Four of the state's educational centers—all important contributors to the cultural, scientific, and technological wealth of our region—have for the first time joined forces formally to present the series. One lecture in the first series was given on the St. Paul campus of the University of Minnesota, one at Carleton College (Dr. Spink's alma mater and a leading liberal arts college), one on the Duluth campus of the university, and one at the Medical School of the university's Minneapolis campus.

Foreword

We are indeed pleased that W. I. B. Beveridge was able to come to Minnesota to present the initial Spink Lectures, which form the basis for this book. In the following chapters, Professor Beveridge provides a glimpse of both the extraordinary breadth and the unfathomable depths of comparative medicine. In the first chapter, we are treated to a historical analysis of comparative medicine and to Professor Beveridge's view of the usefulness in historic perspective of analogy as a method of research in medicine and biology. While accepting certain limitations of analogy in logical and scientific pursuits, Professor Beveridge points to the importance of models of human disease especially as these occur naturally in the study of animal disease. He has been able to trace to the influence of comparative medicine many key steps in the development of the concepts of contagion, etiological agents, vectors of disease, wind transmission of virus infection, and vaccination involving both live virus vaccines and killed organism vaccines. His considerations carry us even to very recent progress in immunizations against parasites and to modern concepts of immunobiology such as those underlying transplant surgery.

Professor Beveridge attributes much of this progress to the understanding of biologic phenomena initially observed and analyzed in animals. He points out that this has been apparent not only in the field of infectious disease but also in work with cancer, where comparative studies have clearly pointed to the association of cancer with virus and to the close relation between endocrine function and the expression of many cancers. Similarly, in cardiovascular and neurological medicine and even in the perplexing area of congenital malformation, Professor Beveridge points out that much has been learned and much more will be learned from comparative studies. He deals as well with the fact that comparative medicine has

11

alerted us—in time, it is to be hoped—to the biologic hazards of pollution and overpopulation, emphasizing that man's very survival may depend on studies of the behavior of his fellow animals.

In the second chapter, Professor Beveridge takes a closer look at many animal models and considers their relevance to successful research using the comparative approach. Breadth of scientific perspective achieved by collaboration may lead to useful results, but it is only second best to breadth within the individual investigator. In this chapter, Professor Beveridge considers the virus etiologies of cancer and congenital anomaly, tissue culture of cells, reverse transcription in carcinogenesis, environmental poisons, autoimmunity, arthritis, immunopathology, and immunization against cancer from the point of view of the comparative pathologist.

Coming to the very specific in his final chapter on the comparative study of influenza, Professor Beveridge demonstrates that through the comparative perspective one can begin to understand the complex genetics of viruses themselves. It is this approach which is leading to an explanation of the new disease variants that arise unpredictably and sweep over the globe as destructive plagues of influenza. He points to convincing evidence that new pandemic strains are produced by the interaction of old human and animal strains. When by chance cells of a human host are doubly infected under just the right circumstances with an animal variant and a human variant, genetic exchange can take place between the two viruses to produce a new and antigenically different strain. This is an exciting new concept that tells why new variants seem to originate frequently in certain areas of Asia where man and his beasts live in close conjunction.

It has been especially interesting to me to reflect on the comparative approach to medical progress espoused by Professor Beveridge and its relationship to the approach to immunobiology my associates and I have been using at Minnesota over the past thirty years.

I was trained in hematology by Hal Downey, a clinical and experimental hematologist who viewed the differentiation of blood cells in a comparative and evolutionary perspective. I further studied extensively in neuroanatomy and physiology with A. T. Rasmussen and Berry Campbell, both of whom had been strongly influenced by the comparative neuroanatomist J. B. Johnston. It thus seems natural that my investigations and those of my students regularly have focused on comparative and evolutionary considerations. Further, I was persuaded to concentrate on clinical medicine by the pediatrician Irvine McQuarrie, who taught and enthusiastically professed that while the business of pediatrics is developmental biology, the best clinical research should represent attempts to interpret in the laboratory the questions generated by "experiments of nature" encountered in the clinic. Thus, through the years we have been trying to understand disease and basic biology through the experimental interpretation of natural clinical phenomena in the light of developmental and comparative considerations. Our approach has yielded numerous exciting and useful results which we have been privileged frequently to return to our patients in the form of new or improved methods of diagnosis and treatment.

Even though at first glance it may seem contradictory to use comparative medicine as a means of gaining critical perspective from which to view clinical issues and to regard the clinic as a point of departure for fundamental studies in comparative biology, the two methods have much in common. The most important similarity, I believe, relates to the regular exposure to questions from multiple perspectives, thus avoiding too narrow a focus. I would anticipate that both approaches will generate much that is useful for man in the years ahead.

In this first series of Spink Lectures, we have been given an example toward which future scholar-lecturers surely must aspire as they reflect further on the potentials of comparative medicine and comparative biology in subsequent contributions to this series.

Robert A. Good

University of Minnesota
May 1972

ACKNOWLEDGMENTS

I wish to express my deep appreciation for the signal honor of being invited to give the first Wesley W. Spink Lectures on Comparative Medicine, which form the basis for this book. It was indeed a rare privilege to inaugurate the lecture series which, over the years to come, is bound to have a far-reaching effect on scientific thinking in its field. It is particularly appropriate that the series is dedicated to a man whose exploration of scientific frontiers has provided splendid examples of the new insights that can be obtained when the study of disease in man is integrated with research on disease in animals.

W. I. B. Beveridge

School of Veterinary Medicine
Cambridge, England
May 1972

Frontiers in Comparative Medicine

INTRODUCTION

Comparative medicine is one of the most exciting fields for scientific work. The horizons of scientists, like those of other men, tend to be restricted by the disciplines of their professional training, so that the weight of research carried out in medical and veterinary studies vastly exceeds that done in the common field. Nevertheless, the modest amount of comparative investigation carried out has already led to a body of discoveries which are fundamental and from which it is clear that the rewards of the comparative method are disproportionately greater than those of either of the two established separate disciplines. Ever since the great work of Charles Darwin, man has been seen to be but one of the animal species, yet the major stream of scientific thinking has continued to proceed on the basis of the old premise of a fundamental division between the human and animal worlds. One consequence of the undervaluation of comparative medicine as a subject is that the methods of research appropriate to it are insufficiently understood, and one of the main purposes of this book is to contribute to the examination of such methods. A whole future of discoveries lies before those of the young generation of scientists who realize sufficiently the potential of the comparative approach to medical and veterinary problems.

In this study I shall take a fresh look at the concept of comparative medicine, treating it as a method in research and first examining just what is involved and how it operates, then showing something of what has been achieved by this method and indicating its potential for the future.

I shall start with some remarks on the logic of analogy as a scientific method and then describe the history of some key discoveries which have demonstrated the value of the comparative method. This will lead to a panoramic view of the scientific fields in which the comparative method is being used at present and will indicate those fields which I believe are particularly favorable for future development. The survey is followed by a description and discussion in more detail of the use of animal models in research on human disease.

The last chapter develops another aspect of comparative medicine by describing the biology of an infectious disease, influenza, which provides a striking illustration of the unity of medicine through the exchange of knowledge and of the agent across species.

CHAPTER 1

THE LOGIC OF THE COMPARATIVE METHOD

O rdinarily we do not reason deliberately following the rules of logic, and we are not consciously aware of what makes our thoughts flow this way or that. I believe that the importance of the part played by analogy in our thinking—scientifically and otherwise—is not sufficiently appreciated. Very commonly our actions are the consequence of our regarding a new situation as analogous to one with which we are familiar.

An analogy is a resemblance between the relationships of things, rather than between the things themselves. When one perceives that the relationship between A and B resembles the relationship between X and Y on one point, and one knows that A is related to B in various other ways, this suggests that one should look for similar relationships between X and Y. Clearly there is no certainty about this sort of reasoning. The value of analogies is that they are suggestive, not that they prove anything, and often they provide the only form of reasoning available. In any case it is as well to remember that in research much of our thinking inevitably is speculative. It is a fallacy to suppose that we can prove a theory in any absolute sense. One can only prove that something happened in the past; a theory must be concerned with past, present, and future if it is to be of any value. The usual procedure in research is to accumulate evidence which more and more people, judging it subjectively, find convincing, until eventually the theory is accepted by practically everyone.

Strictly speaking, comparative medicine means comparing disease phenomena in different species, including man, but in the present discussion I regard it as meaning research by analogy between disease in man, on the one hand, and disease in the rest of the animal kingdom, on the other. When we see that an animal disease and a human disease have certain characteristics in common, we are led to think they may have also other characteristics in common. Having recognized that the clinical and pathological manifestations of the two diseases are similar, we reason by analogy that if we can find out more about the animal disease, the knowledge so gained can be applied to the human problem. This is the logic behind using animal models in medical research.

However, this bare outline may lead to an oversimplified view which can give rise to misunderstandings. Comparative medicine usually involves more than just taking results obtained in research with animals and applying them directly to the human problem, that is to say, extrapolating them. Research on animals enables general principles to be discerned, and it is these that are transferred to the study of the human problem. By "general principles" I mean theoretical concepts, understanding of the physicochemical mechanisms involved, and the development of technical methods. To put it another way, comparative medicine indicates what we should look for in man and how to go about it.

In practice, the comparative method may be more complex

than it appears in retrospect when the problem can be seen clearly. Sometimes the problem is to find meaningful analogues, that is, models. There may be no difficulty with clear-cut situations, such as an infectious disease or nutritional deficiency disease, if it occurs naturally in some other species as well as in man. With some human diseases, however, it is difficult to find an analogous condition in an animal, or the difficulty may be to decide whether a disease in an animal is sufficiently similar to be a useful model. In such situations there is much scope for personal judgments and consequently for differences of opinion.

I do not wish to suggest that the advances in comparative medicine are always due to research planned in advance. Many discoveries have been made in the course of investigations carried out on diseases of domestic animals because of the economic importance of those diseases, without any intention of throwing light on human diseases, and only subsequently was it found that the new knowledge could be transferred to analogous human diseases. In comparative medicine, as in most fields of research, new knowledge is won in either of two ways: by a planned effort to solve a recognized problem or by opportunism, that is, seizing on an unexpected finding and following up its implications.

Origin of New Concepts of Communicable Disease

I shall give some examples of discoveries made in animals which have had far-reaching effects on human medicine. In order to understand the significance of a discovery, it is necessary to know something of the problem as it appeared before the discovery was made. Let us look at the general problem of the nature and cause of infectious diseases, seen in its most blatant form in great epidemics. A vague idea that they were due in some way to transmission of some mysterious agent had been current since biblical times, but it was not looked on favorably by the medical profession and competed with hypotheses about spirits and the wrath of the gods and about the influence of the stars and comets. The concept of contagion as something that spread from person to person and from town to town during an epidemic became fairly widely accepted during the Middle Ages, largely as a result of epidemics of the great plague. But the nature of the contagion itself remained vague—it was loosely thought of as a chemical property of the air, something like a bad smell. Thinking on the subject was greatly clarified by the Italian Girolamo Fracastoro in the middle of the sixteenth century. He likened contagion to the spread of rot from one apple to another in contact with it and spoke of seeds or germs of disease which propagate other germs exactly like themselves. But the effect of this brilliant insight was somewhat limited by the general belief (held also by Fracastoro) that these germs could arise spontaneously within people or in the air or earth. After enjoying a short-lived popularity, his teaching was largely forgotten. As has so often happened, the growth of knowledge was held up by widely accepted erroneous beliefs which first had to be cleared up. Belief in spontaneous generation and heterogenesis had to be overcome before the way was open for the establishment of the basic facts about the germ theory of disease.

The last hundred years or so have been the golden age of conquest of communicable diseases. We can learn much about how knowledge grows by looking into the way the breakthroughs have been made, so I shall describe briefly some of the key discoveries.

The first time that a microbe was shown to be the cause of

a disease of any animal was in 1834 when the Italian Agostino Bassi demonstrated that a disease of silkworms known as "calcino" was due to a particular fungus. He showed that the disease could not arise spontaneously, that it could be transmitted experimentally, and that the infectious agent could be destroyed by certain chemicals, thus establishing foundations for research on other communicable diseases. Although educated in law and employed as a civil servant, Agostino Bassi has been acknowledged as the first to provide firm evidence in support of the hypothesis that infectious diseases are caused by living microbes.

Bassi's work led to a search for microbes in communicable diseases of man and animals. The next landmark was the discovery of the bacillus which causes anthrax in sheep. The discovery was made in about 1850 by Casimir Davaine in France and Franz Pollender in Germany. The "germ theory of disease," as it then came to be called, attracted much attention, but most authorities refused to accept that there was a true analogy between anthrax in sheep and infectious diseases in man, or, as we would say now, they did not see the sheep disease as a model for infectious diseases of man. Fortunately there were some pioneers who followed up the implications of this discovery. Yet it was not until about 1880 that the work of Louis Pasteur, Robert Koch, and others on anthrax commanded general acceptance of the germ theory. It is hard to believe that this was less than a hundred years ago—within one lifetime.

The next microbes found to cause disease were the blood-inhabiting protozoans, the trypanosomes. T. R. Lewis found them in the blood of rats in 1878, but the significant advance came in 1897 when David Bruce reported that his research had proved trypanosomes to be the cause of a disease of cattle in Africa called nagana. It was five years later that trypanosomes were shown to be the cause of sleeping sickness in man.

However, it was soon found that there were many contagious diseases in which microbes visible with the light microscope could not be demonstrated. The next landmark was the discovery of viruses. Working in Germany, Friedrich Loeffler and Paul Frosch found that foot-and-mouth disease of cattle could be transmitted by a bacteria-free filtrate. At about the same time, a disease of tobacco plants was also found to be transmissible in this way. The concept of the so-called "ultravisible, filtrable viruses" was thus born in 1898. This led within the next few years to yellow fever and other human diseases being shown to be due to the microbes which we now call simply viruses.

Another group of organisms was also discovered around the turn of the century during investigations on a disease of cattle. Nocard, Roux, and Dujardin-Beaumetz isolated the first Mycoplasma from cases of contagious bovine pleuropneumonia. Curiously, there was a delay of fifty years before it was shown that a Mycoplasma also causes pneumonia in man.

This is still not the end of the remarkable series of discoveries of pathogenic microbes. A completely different and as yet little understood type of infectious agent was found to cause that curious, slowly developing, nervous disease of sheep known as scrapie. The nature of this agent is still largely a mystery. It has not been possible to visualize it under the electron microscope and, more remarkable, it seems to have no nucleic acid. One theory is that scrapie activity is due to an assemblage of macromolecules bound in a membrane complex. I shall mention the extension of this work to human problems later in this chapter.

This completes the series of infectious agents—fungi, bacteria, trypanosomes, Mycoplasma, viruses, scrapie-like agents

—discovered in the course of investigations on diseases of animals. Next let us look at the way these manage to get from one host to the next. It had long been suspected that arthropods—insects, ticks, mites—were in some way involved in the cause of a number of diseases, but this was only a vague hypothesis until about 1890, when Frederick Kilborne showed experimentally that Texas fever of cattle was transmitted from host to host by ticks. Subsequently, the vital role of arthropod vectors was demonstrated in malaria and many other diseases of man and animals.

During the last decade or so, it has been found that two highly infectious diseases of domestic animals—foot-and-mouth disease of cattle and Newcastle disease of chickens—are sometimes spread by the wind over distances of several miles. So far there has been no evidence that the human diseases actually do spread in this way, but it is a grim warning of what could happen if the hounds of hell were unleashed in biological warfare.

The reason why the word "vaccine," derived from the Latin *vaccinus*, a cow, is used as a general term for immunizing agents is that the concept originated from Edward Jenner's pioneering work on immunization against smallpox in the latter part of the eighteenth century. Historical accounts of this discovery often give the impression that it simply arose from Jenner's casual observation that milkmaids who had had cowpox did not get smallpox. This is an oversimplification. The truth is that Jenner made a detailed study of pox diseases in cows, horses, and pigs; he was in fact using the comparative medicine approach to smallpox. Cowpox is only one of several diseases found on cows' teats and on milkers' hands, and it was because Jenner had studied the problem that he was able to select the appropriate material from cows to use for vaccination against smallpox.

Eighty years passed before the next breakthrough. Then Louis Pasteur discovered how to immunize fowls against fowl cholera by inoculating them with a living attenuated culture of the causal bacterium. He established the principle that a vaccine can be made by reducing the virulence of the causal organism in the laboratory, and this method was soon applied to anthrax, rabies, and many other diseases of man and animals.

The next development was vaccines made from killed organisms. Realization that this was possible originated from the investigations of Daniel Salmon and Theobald Smith on swine plague in 1886. They isolated a bacterium, cultures of which killed pigeons on inoculation. They tried to show that the cultures contained a toxin by heating them just sufficiently to kill the bacteria and then inoculating them into pigeons. They were disappointed when the birds showed no reaction, but when two of the same birds were inoculated with live culture eighteen days later, they were found to be immune. This was the origin of the concept of killed vaccines, which have since been used to protect men and animals against many diseases.

Until recently, no one had been successful in producing a vaccine that would protect against worm parasites. However, within the last fifteen years at the Glasgow Veterinary School, a group of veterinarians headed by William Jarrett have learned how to immunize cattle against lungworm. The method also works with hookworm, and work is now in progress which will probably result in a vaccine to protect people from hookworm.

The modern developments in transplant surgery in man were made possible by the discovery of the principle of immunological tolerance. This stems from an observation in animals. It concerns twin calves whose placentas had fused and hence their fetal blood had mixed. Each twin was found to retain some cells from the other throughout life: in other words they were tolerant to cells that were not their own, which no animal or person normally is.

Just within the last year or so, we have seen the successful development and widespread application of the first vaccine against a cancer. I refer to the vaccine against Marek's disease of chickens. There are in fact three different vaccines, each made from a nonpathogenic strain of the causal virus. The way in which these vaccines confer protection is not yet understood, but it seems to differ fundamentally from the way that other virus vaccines work.

So we see that in the fields of infectious diseases and immunology most of the key discoveries were made during the course of investigations on animal disease. Probably these are the fields where the greatest number of key discoveries have originated in animals, but very many have also been made with animals in other fields, especially in nutrition and genetics. I think enough examples have been given to show that the principles of disease can be revealed more readily in animals than in man, and it is worth looking into the reasons for this.

I suggest there are four reasons. The first is that farm animals are kept under control in the following ways: (a) they are either restricted to certain grazing areas or are kept indoors in large numbers and fed on imposed man-made diets; (b) they are subjected to husbandry practices that are different from those under which they evolved; and (c) they are selectively bred for rapid growth and high production, often with a degree of inbreeding. In short, man has created an artificial biological situation in which disease problems are likely to arise or be accentuated.

The second reason is that most animals have a relatively

short life span and are kept in groups under constant supervision; hence, problems are more easily recognized. Efficiency of production is a very sensitive indicator of health.

The third and most important reason is that experimental procedures and intervention studies are feasible in animals that are not permissible in man. Investigations are not handicapped by reverence for the life and welfare of each sick individual. Pathological studies in man are confined largely to the terminal stages of a disease, whereas study of the pathology in the early stages is usually more informative.

Finally, I would add a fourth factor, the socioeconomic one. Under conditions of modern intensive animal production, disease—even a mild disease—adversely affects the economy of the enterprise and hence cannot be tolerated; every effort must be made to prevent it and to maintain as perfect a state of health as possible. By contrast, in man there has been a tendency to accept a degree of suboptimal health as beyond our control, and the individual is free to overindulge himself in ways that are often deleterious to his health.

Some Current Developments and Future Prospects

Infectious diseases are no longer the main causes of death in the advanced countries. Their place has been taken by the degenerative diseases, especially cardiovascular disease and cancer. It is worth noting that research on animal diseases has been concentrated on communicable diseases because they are the ones that have been economically important. This partly explains why there has been so much "spin off " in this field, whereas there has been little so far in the degenerative diseases which have attracted less research in animals. These economically unimportant diseases in animals must be studied with the deliberate intention of using them as models for human diseases, and today this is being done to an ever-increasing extent. I shall describe briefly the work going on in some of the more important fields.

CANCER

Let us first look at cancer. This is the subject on which probably more comparative studies have been done than any other and where the most important results have been obtained. The first demonstration that some tumors may be transferred from one animal to another took place nearly a hundred years ago. It was in 1876 that the Russian veterinarian M. A. Novinsky succeeded in transplanting venereal sarcoma from dog to dog. The discovery that some cancers are caused by viruses was announced over sixty years ago. The American Peyton Rous showed in 1910 that a sarcoma of a breast muscle could be transmitted to other chickens by a cell-free and bacteria-free filtrate. Since then viruses have been shown to be the cause of many other neoplastic conditions in a wide variety of animals—including cold-blooded species, birds, and a number of mammalian species. In 1969 it was said that eighty viruses were known which cause cancer in every major group of animals including nonhuman primates. But despite intensive experimental investigations over a number of years, until recently the skeptics were able to say that, although of great scientific interest, this work was probably not applicable to human problems. Like many other aspects of cancer research, the problems have been found to be extremely complex. Most discoveries have only limited implications for other situations and other species, instead of revealing fundamental principles with wide application.

Quite recently the picture has changed. Herpes-type viruses have been shown to cause Marek's disease of chickens, a lymphoma in certain monkeys, and probably adenoma of the lungs of sheep. Similar viruses have been found in a lymphoma of children in Africa known as Burkitt's tumor, in nasopharyngeal cancer in Chinese, and in the cancer of the uterine cervix of women which is common throughout the world. The causal significance of the virus in these human cancers is not yet proved, but there is considerable circumstantial evidence for it, backed by the analogy with the animal tumors. There is also suggestive evidence of a virus in breast cancer in women. Apart from the work with viruses, many other aspects of cancer in animals are being studied. Epidemiological studies show that there are enormous differences in the frequency with which various types of cancer occur naturally in different localities, different species, different breeds, and different organs. There is unlimited scope for investigation to discover the reasons for these differences. These studies involve physiology, especially hormones, and various aspects of the environment, especially the food. So far there has been only a limited amount of work done in this field, but some useful results have emerged. Substances occurring naturally in certain plants, such as bracken, and in certain fungi infecting their feed have been shown to cause cancer in animals. There is suggestive evidence that these substances may account for unusually high incidence of cancer in people in particular regions. Also there have been instances where food additives have been found to cause cancer in animals.

Animals are also valuable for investigating new methods of treating cancer. Several types of cancer can be produced experimentally in rodents, thus providing experimental animal models for therapeutic trials. This means that cancer research workers are able to use comparable groups of animals, a tool which provided the basis for so much fruitful research on infectious diseases and nutritional diseases. However, for some types of investigation rodents are too small, and tumor-bearing dogs and monkeys are required for trying out techniques before applying them to man. Two types of tumor can be produced readily in monkeys and in dogs, and special techniques have been developed whereby several types of cancer can be transplanted in dogs. Apart from therapeutic trials, dogs and monkeys are also valuable for research on immunology of cancer.

CARDIOVASCULAR DISEASES

The second group of degenerative diseases that have become such an increasingly important cause of ill health and death in advanced countries comprises the cardiovascular diseases. The number one problem is, of course, atherosclerosis, which underlies most heart deaths and strokes. The most striking fact to note at the start is that atherosclerosis does not constitute a problem in domestic or wild animals. It does occur, but the lesions seldom become severe enough to cause overt illness or death.

When the World Health Organization sought to encourage and coordinate comparative studies in this field ten years ago, we did not have good models readily at hand as there were with cancer, and the first need was to carry out surveys in as many species as possible to ascertain which was the most suitable for this type of research. Mild lesions of atherosclerosis were found in many species. The animals in which the lesions were best developed and most similar histologically to those in man were found to be certain monkeys, especially Cebus and squirrel monkeys, pigs, and some birds such as pigeons and chickens. These animals have since been used in various experiments to determine the effect of diet and social stress on heart disease.

Results of considerable interest have been obtained in experiments on social stress in chickens and in pigs carried out by Dr. Herbert Ratcliffe in Philadelphia. In the chickens there was little or no disease of the arteries in groups consisting of either all males or all females, but in groups made up of twice as many males as females there was much arterial disease and a number of heart deaths. Experiments of a similar nature in pigs also showed that in some social situations animals developed more lesions than those in other situations. The lesions were worst in individuals in solitary confinement, intermediate in animals kept as pairs, and least in the animals kept in groups. These results may not have direct application to the human situation, but they provide objective evidence of the general principle that psychological factors do play a role in cardiovascular disease, and they provide models with which a critical analysis can be made of the physiological factors involved. Ultimately such studies could well throw light on human problems.

NEUROPATHOLOGY

A wide variety of diseases of the central nervous system occur in animals. Some of these are counterparts of the human diseases, and some are in fact transferrable between man and animal. The classical example is rabies. Some virus infections of the brain of man and animals are transmitted by insects and other arthropods. The first viral encephalitis shown to be transmitted in this way was encephalomyelitis of horses.

Today there are still a number of slowly developing degenerative diseases of the brain of man, the causes of which are unknown or imperfectly understood. Research in diseases of this type in animals has brought to light new knowledge which is now being used to study these very difficult problems in man. The most intriguing investigations are those on the sheep disease scrapie, which I mentioned earlier as being caused by a transmissible agent that seems to have no nucleic acid. Progress in research on this disease has been slow, partly because the incubation period in sheep lasts for years—therefore each experiment took a long time—and partly because of the technical difficulties of working with an agent which is resistant to disinfectants and prolonged boiling. Progress has been more rapid during the past few years, after it was found that the disease could be transmitted to mice, in which the incubation period is only a matter of months.

The next important development was the discovery that a comparable disease occurs in mink. The long incubation period, the pathology, and the properties of the infectious agent are essentially similar to those of scrapie. The knowledge gained from scrapie has been applied successfully to investigations on two human brain diseases known as kuru and Jakob-Creutzfeldt disease. These two human diseases resemble the sheep and mink disease in that when they are transmitted experimentally they have an incubation period of many months, the clinical picture is that of a progressive fatal disease of the central nervous system, and on autopsy the pathology is similar. The transmissible agent cannot be detected by electron microscopy or by presently available tissue culture or immunological techniques. There is suggestive evidence that at least one other more common nervous disease of man—disseminated sclerosis—may have affinities with these diseases.

New concepts arising out of research on scrapie and allied conditions are leading to reconsideration of the possibility of an infectious etiology of a number of diseases which have been regarded as genetic or immunopathological disorders. Further, scrapie involves pathological changes in the brain that have been likened to a speeding up of the aging process. Could this observation provide a starting point for a new line of investigation into the nature of aging and various degenerative processes associated with it?

CONGENITAL MALFORMATIONS

Congenital malformations have assumed increasing importance in medically advanced countries. There are two reasons. Firstly, neonatal deaths due to infectious and deficiency diseases have been greatly reduced, but deaths due to malformations have not been reduced to the same extent; so malformations are now a leading cause of mortality in the newborn. Secondly, there is an increase in the proportion of malformed babies surviving; some of these remain permanently handicapped.

In the area of veterinary medicine, many of the animals that are obviously abnormal at birth soon die from lack of special care or are deliberately destroyed as unwanted. Nevertheless, there are many congenital defects diagnosed in patients at veterinary clinics. In one survey involving over a hundred thousand domestic animals, nearly 5 percent were diagnosed as having congenital abnormalities. Some of the more common defects were cryptorchism, hip dysplasia, dislocation of the patella, eye and lid defects, hernias, malformations of the heart and great vessels, hydrocephalus, contracted tendons, defects of the penis and prepuce, hypoplasia of the cerebellum, imperforate anus, deafness, and cleft palate.

Disease of the fetus may lead either to its death, with consequent abortion or stillbirth, or else to malformation. Fetal pathology is a very broad field encompassing practically all the biomedical sciences—genetics, nutrition, infectious diseases, pharmacology, physiology, and many others. There are many well-known animal models of human problems in this area, and the survey just mentioned suggests there is probably still plenty of scope for further comparative studies here.

The Logic of the Comparative Method

Other fields where comparative studies have much to contribute to human well-being are environmental pollution and problems due to overpopulation. Fortunately, many governments have realized recently the enormous problems mankind is creating for itself by mutilating and polluting our environment, consequent on the population explosion and massive industrialization. In this devastation, the first to suffer are the plants and animals. By observing them, we can sometimes see in advance what will happen to man unless something is done to check the irresponsible rape of our beautiful planet.

Toxic residues derived from industrial wastes or pesticides can often be detected in various animals. Fortunately for us, some mammals, birds, and fishes are more sensitive to many of these than is man, and careful monitoring can often warn us of the dangers. Using sentinel animals to monitor the environment is by no means a new idea. In the last century the miner's canary was used to warn against dangerous atmospheric conditions in mines and sewers.

Most thinking people and governments are now conscious of the terrible problems threatening mankind from excessive population. Here again there is much we can learn from animals. Back in 1798, Thomas Malthus postulated that populations of people and animals are kept in check by famine and disease. We now know that this is by no means the whole story. Many species have evolved methods of limiting their reproduction rate to about that necessary to maintain the population at the level which the living space can support. These methods of population limitation take the form of social behavioral patterns, sometimes linked with the physiology of reproduction of the species. They can be observed where man has not disturbed the natural ecological balance. Comparative medicine has helped greatly in the development of methods of reducing human mortality from communicable disease and malnutrition, indirectly leading to the population explosion; perhaps we can also learn something from animals on how to check excessive growth of the human population.

MENTAL HEALTH

I have kept until the last comments on a field in which I believe we will see, in the not too distant future, developments of greater importance for the happiness of mankind than in all other aspects of medicine. Progress in investigations on degenerative disease has been slow, but even slower has been progress toward understanding and preventing mental illness and neuroses of all sorts and toward solving sociological problems associated with our civilization. In the Western world today, there probably is more suffering and unhappiness caused by mental troubles than by physical disease.

The difference between us and other animals is due to the knowledge we have accumulated over the last ten thousand years, not to any fundamental biological change that has taken place in the few hundred generations since the beginning of civilization. Our species evolved and adapted to an environment and way of life very different from those found in modern civilization. It is not surprising that many individuals are unable to adjust themselves successfully to the complexities of modern life for which evolution has ill-prepared them. Only by understanding the animal within us and the way it influences our behavior can we understand ourselves and learn to cope with the problems arising therefrom.

Until recently, our thinking has been obscured by the widely held traditional conviction that man is a being quite apart from the rest of the animal kingdom. Not only did the Christian religion assert that man alone has a soul, but many psychologists held that consciousness is something that only man experiences. The barrier broken a century or more ago regarding physical diseases is only now being overcome in the mental field.

Comparative studies in behavior started with Charles Darwin, but the modern era started only about thirty years ago. The last decade has seen a revolution in the behavioral sciences, the far-reaching implications of which only now are becoming generally realized. Many behavioral patterns which had long been regarded as characteristically "human" have been found firmly established and innate in other species, often amazingly far down the evolutionary tree. A sense of possession of territory and of home, a sense of social status, loyalty to one's group and cooperation in defense in the face of outside threats, distrust of strangers and outsiders, responsibility toward one's mate and one's offspring: when my behavior or yours is governed by these considerations, we are obeying the same laws as are written into the genetic code of most vertebrates. Just as a large proportion of the genes that built our bodies are shared with many mammals, so also are those that built our minds. Can it be doubted that divided loyalties and conflicting desires that worry us also worry animals? Abnormal behavioral patterns do occur occasionally in animals.

Extensive studies in normal and abnormal behavior of animals are being undertaken today. Through ethology, at last an experimental method has been found for studying psychological problems and mental disease. Is it unreasonable to expect an explosion of knowledge comparable to that which followed the demonstration of the germ theory of disease? I believe that it is here that we shall see the most revolutionary developments in medicine during the working lifetime of those who are students today. The leaders will be scientists with a broad biological outlook who are able to recognize the analogies between the animal model systems and the human problems and to use the comparative approach. They will be men with "prepared minds," to borrow Louis Pasteur's phrase, men whose mental background enables them to perceive the parallel between familiar things and the only partly known, as Isaac Newton did with the falling apple and the moon. William Blake, with poetic insight, reveals the power of analogy in these words:

> *To see a world in a grain of sand,*
> *And a heaven in a wild flower;*
> *Hold infinity in the palm of your hand,*
> *And eternity in an hour.*

CHAPTER 2

ANIMAL MODELS
OF HUMAN DISEASES

I n the preceding chapter, I pointed out that the logic behind comparative medicine is that of doing research by
analogy, and I outlined in general terms some of the fields in
which this method has been successfully used. In this chapter, I shall look more closely at some model systems. First,
however, I shall consider the ways in which suitable models
for human problems are found.

Basically, there are two approaches to the discovery of such
models: starting from the animal or starting from man. In
the first case, someone working with animals, usually a veterinarian, notices that an animal disease which he encounters
resembles a human disease which he knows about, and he
draws attention to the possible value of the former as a model
for the latter. Clearly, the recognition of these opportunities
depends on the veterinarian being acquainted with human
pathology. In the second case, the researcher starts from the
human disease and makes a deliberate search for an analogous
condition in animals. Here, again, it is necessary for the person concerned to have some knowledge of both human and

animal disease in order to draw analogies which have significant implications for further research.

The first point I wish to make, then, is that comparative medicine calls for research workers whose knowledge is broader than normally met in people trained exclusively in either the veterinary or the medical field. Veterinary education always extends across several species of animals, so usually it is easier for the veterinarian to acquire a general knowledge of human diseases than it is for a medical man to acquire knowledge of diseases of animals. It might be argued that collaboration between a medic and a veterinarian renders it unnecessary for either to know the other's field, but this is only partly true, and, in my view, it is a second best to combining the knowledge in one mind. Dependence on collaboration lessens the chance of unforeseen discovery. Whichever way one looks at it, however, it is necessary to bridge the gap that normally exists between human and veterinary medicine.

Animal models are most often found in domestic animals and especially the companion animals, dogs and cats, because they are often kept to old age and given more individual veterinary attention than farm animals. The next most fruitful source is laboratory animals, because they are usually autopsied. Animals in zoos are another source of models and, no doubt, there is a great potential in wild animals, among which, however, there are practical difficulties in finding models. Lower vertebrates and invertebrates also offer scope for comparative studies, and one recalls that the concept of phagocytic cells as part of our defense mechanism originated from Metchnikoff's observation on starfish larvae.

Once a few animals are found with the disease in question, it is sometimes possible to breed from them selectively to produce groups of animals for experimentation and even to intensify the disease condition. Inbreeding of mice has been extensively practiced to produce strains which are especially suitable for studying certain diseases. For example, the New Zealand black mouse is a well-known model in immunopathology.

An animal model may be a true counterpart to the human disease, and in that case direct comparisons and transfer of information can take place; but often the best model that is available differs from the human condition in a number of respects, and this situation calls for careful judgment and insight in interpreting the comparisons. In these cases, it is especially important to bear in mind that the object of the study is not so much to transfer results directly from animal to man as to reach an understanding of the underlying mechanisms of the particular disease in the relevant physiological context. That is why a model may be useful even when it is not an exact counterpart. The essence of the comparative method is that one uses the animal model to elucidate the basic disease processes and to develop appropriate technical methods. One then employs this knowledge to investigate the human problem.

Virtually any medical problem can be approached in the comparative way. Leader and Leader (1971), Jones (1969), Cornelius (1969), and others have produced extensive catalogues of animal models of human diseases. The National Academy of Sciences publishes a series entitled *Animal Models for Biomedical Research,* and the Institute of Laboratory Animal Resources includes details of animal models in the *ILAR News* starting with Volume 13, January 1970. A registry of comparative pathology has been operating at the Armed Forces Institute of Pathology in Washington since 1966. Therefore it would be pointless for me to produce here a long list of models or even cite examples in all the fields. To illustrate the potentialities of comparative medicine, I shall choose a few fields where the most exciting developments are now taking place. In the preceding chapter I described the great contributions made by comparative medicine to the solution of problems of infectious disease. That golden age lies behind us. I shall try to choose fields where the golden age is with us or still lies ahead.

The first I select is cancer research, because there is an explosion of knowledge now going on in this field. The second is immunopathology, which is a relatively young and rapidly developing discipline. The third is environmental pollution, the importance of which is, at last, apparent to everyone. The fourth is congenital malformations, an area in which the great potentialities of the comparative approach have not been sufficiently recognized. The fifth and last is reproduction and population control, a subject which I believe will, in the long run, have a greater influence on the welfare of man and animals than all the rest.

Cancer

These studies have been directed mainly toward arriving at an understanding of the nature and basic cause of neoplasia as a biological phenomenon. The particular aspect which has been most actively pursued is the role of viruses. Viral oncology has become a subject in its own right and has been concerned almost entirely with animal models, although the work has been financed and undertaken with the objective of finding applications in human cancer.

Early hopes that some of the results obtained with animal models would be found to be applicable to human cancer have not, so far, been fulfilled. A wide range of tumors in many animal species have been shown to be caused by viruses, but, surprisingly, there is as yet no clear evidence of a virus causing a cancer in the species we are most interested in—man. The production of cancer by viruses and the detection of viruses in the tumors which they have produced have proved to be a most complicated matter.

Oncogenic RNA viruses are called oncornaviruses or leukoviruses. They cause cancer under natural conditions in chickens, rodents, cats, and certain monkeys. Most of these cancers are leukemias or sarcomas, but in the mammary gland of mice carcinomas are produced. Generally speaking, infection with these viruses is extremely common, but only a relatively small proportion of the infected animals develop cancer naturally. Oncornaviruses multiply readily in appropriate cell cultures; usually they do not kill the cells, but in some instances they transform them, that is, the cells take on the characteristics of malignant cells. Often infective virus is not produced in the cell cultures because the virus is "defective"; such a virus can be "rescued" by simultaneous infection of the cell with a related "helper" virus which provides the missing parts. In the tumors caused by oncornaviruses, the virus can be demonstrated by electron microscopy and often by serological tests and isolation.

This very brief outline of the behavior of oncornaviruses rather oversimplifies the situation, but, broadly speaking, it is correct. The main point to note is that the intact virus genome persists in the tumors and can be detected by the various sophisticated technical methods which have been developed.

If we turn now to oncogenic DNA viruses, we find that the position is different and even more involved, at least so far as the papovaviruses and the adenoviruses are concerned, certain members of which have been shown to be capable of producing cancer under laboratory conditions. Most of the papovaviruses and adenoviruses rarely, if ever, produce tumors in

45

nature, but they do readily when inoculated into the newborn rodents. In cell cultures, they transform the cells, which thereupon acquire certain antigens specific for the virus, called "T" (for tumor) antigens. The remarkable thing is that these antigens are produced in each succeeding generation of cells, but the intact virus genome does not persist. Fragments of the virus genome are integrated with the cell's DNA, making up about 1/5,000th of the total DNA in the cell, and these pieces of virus replicate with the cell's genome. The effect is that about 2 percent of messenger RNA in the cell is virus-coded. Therefore, to detect that a tumor has been caused by a papovavirus or adenovirus requires even more sophisticated technical methods than with tumors caused by the oncornaviruses, where the whole virus genome is perpetuated.

A tremendous amount of very fundamental work has been devoted to working out the complexities of virus-cell interactions and the molecular biology of the oncornaviruses, papovaviruses, and adenoviruses, and to using the systems as models to investigate certain human cancers, particularly leukemia and mammary cancer. As I have said, for many years there was little to show so far as results with man are concerned, but at last there seems to be a breakthrough. Moore and his colleagues (1971) in Camden (New Jersey), Detroit, and Bombay reported finding B-type virus particles in milk from a number of women whose relatives had breast cancer.

To understand the background of this recent finding, we must go back some sixty years. It was Murray who first recognized that mammary cancer in mice was a useful model of mammary cancer in women. He undertook breeding experiments which showed that certain families of mice had a higher incidence than others (Murray, 1911). It was generally believed that the familial high incidence was due to genetic predisposition until, in 1936, Bittner showed it was due to

46

transmission of some unknown factor in the mother's milk (Bittner, 1936). This so-called "Bittner milk factor" was eventually shown to be an oncornavirus, i.e., an RNA virus with a unique morphology referred to as B-type. A great deal of research was devoted to this topic, since the mouse cancer appeared to be a good model for human breast cancer—one of the most prevalent and serious human cancers. The similarities between the mouse and human disease are striking. The overall incidence rate in women and in wild mice is roughly the same, and in both species there is a high rate in certain families. Both are adenocarcinomas.

Recently Moore and his colleagues examined the milk of women with a history of breast cancer in their families as opposed to that of women whose relatives did not have breast cancer. They found the characteristic B-type particles in about half of the former and only one-twentieth of the latter. Further, Charney and Moore (1971) obtained some suggestive evidence that women with breast cancer may have antibodies which react against an antigen of the mouse virus, though the results so far published are by no means conclusive. The identity of the B-type particles in the human milk as RNA virus was later confirmed by Schlom, Spiegelman, and Moore (1971). They found that milk with these particles contained reverse transcriptase, that is, RNA-dependent DNA polymerase, whereas milk without the particles did not. So far this enzyme has been found in all thirty-one oncogenic RNA viruses examined and not in other viruses, so its presence in human milk can be taken as contributory evidence, though not proof, that human breast cancer is caused by a virus of this group. Another significant piece of research that fits into this jigsaw puzzle is that a virus similar in many respects to the mouse mammary cancer virus has been isolated from a mammary carcinoma in a rhesus monkey (Chopra and Mason, 1970).

So now, sixty years after Murray's pioneering studies, we are witnessing an exciting stage of the investigation of human breast cancer, based on knowledge gained from study of the animal model. Further developments are eagerly awaited, but many people feel that it is probably only a matter of time before the cause of this most important human cancer will be established. There will, undoubtedly, be implications concerning prevention and treatment, and in developing these the mouse model will be invaluable.

The discovery of Moore and his colleagues is only one of the exciting recent developments in viral oncology. The oncornaviruses, the papovaviruses, and the adenoviruses are not the only ones known to cause cancer in animals; the herpes group is also involved. It is now generally accepted that a herpes-type virus causes carcinoma of the kidney of the leopard frog, Marek's disease of chickens, lymphomas in certain monkeys, and probably pulmonary adenomatosis in sheep. In man, herpes-type viruses are associated with Burkitt's lymphoma, carcinoma of the cervix uteri, and nasopharyngeal carcinoma in Chinese. It is not yet proved that the virus is the causal agent of these three human tumors; it could be merely a passenger, but this seems unlikely.

Marek's disease of chickens is a widespread and economically important neoplastic disease in which lymphoid accumulations occur in various organs, including the nerve trunks, and frequently lead to paralysis. In 1968, Churchill, Biggs, and their colleagues in England showed that it was caused by a herpes virus and later achieved the important step of developing a vaccine that protected chickens against the disease. Improved vaccines have since been produced. During 1971, tens of millions of chickens were vaccinated with excellent results. It is significant that protection conferred by the vaccine seems to be due to different mechanisms from those involved in protection against ordinary viral diseases. Although the vaccine protects against tumors, it does not prevent infection and multiplication of virulent wild virus or its being shed (Eidson *et al.*, 1972). Apparently new principles may be involved in immunization against cancer.

Not only are the vaccines against Marek's disease remarkably safe and effective, but they have yielded an unexpected bonus: they reduce deaths due to other diseases. The explanation is that the Marek's virus not only causes tumors but also depresses the functioning of the immune system, even in those chicks which do not develop tumors, and the vaccine protects against this happening.

The successful development of the first vaccine against a neoplastic disease is undoubtedly a breakthrough of great importance. It is a milestone on the road to cancer prevention that justifies the faith of those workers who have asserted that vaccination against cancer is not just a dream.

Immunopathology

Although in most circumstances immunological processes are beneficial in that they protect us from infection, sometimes these same processes are harmful and cause tissue damage. In certain diseases, particularly those referred to as connective tissue diseases, the main lesions are caused by immune reactions directed against the host's own tissues. In autoimmunity, the defense forces of the body, for some unknown reason, partly lose the restraints which normally prevent them from attacking their own tissues. Rheumatoid arthritis and systemic lupus erythematosus (SLE) are the most important connective tissue diseases, but there are also a number of other conditions in which immunopathology is involved, including some forms of glomerulonephritis and hemolytic anemia. Research has made little progress in elucidating the pathogenesis of these diseases, and the cause or causes are, for the most part, as obscure as with cancer. Indeed, there are similarities in the ways in which research is developing in these two fields.

Several animal diseases are known in which immunopathological lesions are prominent, and these provide an opportunity for detailed analysis of the factors concerned in the pathogenesis of this type of disease. The main ones are systemic lupus and hemolytic anemia of New Zealand black mice and their hybrids, systemic lupus in dogs, Aleutian disease of mink, feline leukemia virus infection in cats, infectious anemia in horses, and lymphocytic choriomeningitis in mice.

The model on which the most research has been done is the disease of New Zealand black mice—NZB, as they are called. This is an inbred strain which rather constantly develops two separate manifestations of autoimmunity, namely, hemolytic anemia and systemic lupus. The lesions mimic fairly closely those seen in man. At first, these conditions were considered to be due to hereditary defects in the animal's immune system and consequently much attention was given to the genetics of the condition by crossing the NZB mice with other strains. Later it was discovered that all NZB mice are infected with a C-type virus, and claims were made that the virus could be transmitted to other mice which then developed the disease. However, these claims have not been substantiated, and the general view at present is that we do not know to what extent the disease is due to the virus or genetic factors. Probably both are involved.

Systemic lupus in dogs also resembles the disease in man and is being studied from hereditary and viral points of view. Some of the progeny of affected parents have developed early signs of the disease, but its distribution is not consistent with any recognized genetic pattern (Lewis and Schwartz, 1971).

This finding and certain other evidence suggest that the disease in dogs may be caused by a virus transmitted vertically in animals which have a genetic susceptibility.

Aleutian disease of mink has definitely been shown to be caused by a virus, but the infection leads to severe disease only in those mink which are homologous for the Aleutian gene that results in a defect in their immunological system. Here we have a clear case of a disease which is only seen in its fully developed form when both a virus and a genetic defect occur together. There is also an example of a virus which not only causes immunopathological lesions but also actually produces a defect in the immune system. Feline leukemia virus inoculated into young kittens destroys the thymus lymphocytes and thus creates an immunodeficient state leading to immunopathological hemolytic anemia and glomerulonephritis (Jarrett, 1972). However, both factors, a virus and an immunological defect, are not always essential for the development of an immunopathological state, because the other two immunopathological models (equine anemia and lymphocytic choriomeningitis in mice) are both caused by viruses, and there does not seem to be any defect in the immune system involved.

The similarity of the pathology in these animal diseases in which viruses are operating and the pathology of systemic lupus and other immunopathological diseases of man has led to an intensive search for viruses in the human counterparts. During the last three years there have been several reports that viruslike particles have been seen by electromicroscopy in affected human tissues (Helder *et al.*, 1971), and efforts are now being made to isolate viruses and determine their etiological significance.

Unfortunately there is no satisfactory animal model for rheumatoid arthritis, the most important of all these diseases, although three or four probable cases have recently been reported in dogs. Attention has been drawn to arthritis in swine due to Erysipelothrix or Mycoplasma, but most rheumatologists do not consider that these conditions provide useful analogies. However, human systemic lupus is in many ways similar to rheumatoid arthritis, and the two conditions sometimes occur in the same patient. If animal models can lead to a solution of the SLE problem, this may in turn throw light on rheumatoid arthritis.

Another disease with some resemblance to rheumatoid arthritis is Reiter's disease of man, in which there is chronic arthritis and immunopathological lesions. Some forms of arthritis in calves, sheep, and pigs have been shown to be caused by Chlamydia, and this finding led to a successful search for Chlamydia in Reiter's disease (Schachter *et al.,* 1966). There is a somewhat similar situation with Mycoplasma, which sometimes causes arthritis in animals and has also been reported as occurring in arthritis in man. The present consensus is that the Chlamydia in Reiter's disease probably plays a causal role, but the significance of the Mycoplasma in human arthritis is doubtful.

I have only touched on one or two points in this rapidly expanding subject. Apart from these advances on the possible role of viruses, the study of animal models has already contributed greatly to our understanding of the basic mechanisms involved in immunopathology (Bulletin of the World Health Organization, 1972).

Environmental Pollution

Except, perhaps, when he lived in the Garden of Eden, man has always been exposed to adverse environmental factors of various kinds: extremes of temperature, the sun's rays, infectious agents, poisons, and so forth. During evolution, man and the other animals have adapted to these natural hazards to a remarkable extent, by genetic variation and natural selection. But since industrialization began, adverse environmental factors have developed abruptly—probably more in the last two hundred years than in the previous ten thousand —and the rate of this development is accelerating alarmingly, so that there is insufficient time for us to adapt genetically to the new exposures. If disastrous consequences are to be avoided, the new man-made factors in the environment must be studied and, where necessary, controlled.

Animals can be used as watchdogs to warn us of danger. For example, aquatic animals have been used as indicators of toxic substances in water. Unpolluted streams, rivers, lakes, and offshore waters normally support a rich variety of animal life, many species of which are extremely sensitive to toxic materials. Therefore, the biologist on the alert is often able to give warning of poisons more easily than the chemist. Many fish and other aquatic animals are being studied in the laboratory to determine their level of sensitivity to various toxic compounds and hence their exact value as sentinel animals.

Farm animals can also be used as watchdogs; for example, when poison gas drifted dangerously on the wind in Utah, warning was given by mortality in sheep. When radioactive fallout occurred accidentally in Britain in 1957, the analysis of cow's milk for radioactive iodine provided a useful measure of the contamination of the environment.

The concept of the food chain has proved of special interest in studies on pollution. Birds of prey, which are at the summit of a food chain, have been seriously affected by DDE, a breakdown product of DDT. Their reproductive rate has fallen drastically because the shells of their eggs have become too fragile. Man is also at the summit of a food chain, so we have to watch not only the toxic substances we are exposed to in air and water, but also those in food, where they may be concentrated. When the sea becomes infested with the poisonous flagellate which gives rise to the phenomenon called the "red tide," the toxin is taken up by shellfish which thereby become poisonous for man. Fortunately for us, the shellfish also become poisonous for birds, and usually mortality in the birds gives warning in time for man to avoid this hazard.

Epidemiological surveillance of domestic and wild animals can be useful in detecting carcinogens, teratogens, and mutagens in the environment. Once again, there are several ways in which animals are of advantage for these studies. Mammals usually spend their entire lives in a restricted area and so are better indicators of localized hazards than man, who moves about so much and is exposed to various environments. There is also the contrasting possibility of using migratory birds to test distant environments. Another advantage of animals is that, with their shorter life span, they develop responses to pollutants in a shorter time than man does. Systematic collection of data on cancer and congenital malformations in animals in relation to locality has seldom been undertaken, but a long-term program has recently been started in Missouri to gather information on congenital malformations in people, pigs, and wild rabbits (Selby *et al.,* 1971).

It has long been known that in certain parts of the world cattle develop bladder cancer. The cause has been found to be a carcinogen in bracken. In some parts of Britain there is a high incidence of stomach cancer in man, and the possibility that this is due to the carcinogen which affects cattle is now being investigated.

Not only can animal studies warn of hazards but sometimes they also lead to unexpected and useful knowledge. A good illustration is the story of moldy sweet clover poisoning in the United States. Investigation of the toxic factor led to the development of a useful anticoagulant for human medicine and the valuable rodenticide, Warfarin. Another illustration is the story of the disease in turkeys which appeared in England a few years ago. This was traced to a particular batch of peanut meal in the feed. Laboratory investigation showed that the meal had been infected with fungus. Eventually the fungus was isolated and the chemistry of the toxin determined, but the story did not end there. The toxin, now known as aflatoxin, was found in small concentrations in many batches of peanuts, and later it was discovered that it caused cancer of the liver in some species. It is known that cancer of the liver occurs with abnormally high frequency in people in parts of Africa, and investigators have found aflatoxin in certain foodstuffs used in Africa. Although it has not yet been established, the suspicion is that the aflatoxin is the cause of the high rate of liver cancer in the people.

These two stories demonstrate the importance and value of undertaking a proper scientific investigation of animal health problems and not merely coping with the immediate practical problems. They also remind us of the important general principle that discovery of knowledge useful to human medicine is not confined to planned studies on recognized models.

Research on the ill effects of pollution is still in an early stage of development. The testing of industrial materials and wastes for possible harmful effects in animals and man is only part of the wider subject of pharmacological and toxicological testing in animals. These tests involve not only drugs and pesticides of all sorts but also the many substances added to foodstuffs as preservatives, flavors, colors, and so on, together with all the other man-made compounds that may contaminate the environment generally. It is said that some half million man-made chemicals are in use today and three thousand new ones are added annually. At present only a few hundred a year are tested in animals. Clearly, there is need for great expansion of testing programs. Substances must be scrutinized not only for acute and chronic toxicity but also for long-term effects such as carcinogenicity, teratogenicity, mutagenicity, and subtle influences on fertility and behavior.

Substances which may have a psychopharmacological effect present a special problem, since we cannot measure subjective effects in animals. Nevertheless, it is feasible to measure a number of behavioral characteristics. In Russia, the conditioned reflex method is being used successfully for detecting early effects of small concentrations of pollutants on the complex functioning of the central nervous system. Animals which have been conditioned to react in certain ways may lose their conditioning when exposed to doses of drugs that have no effect detectable by other means (Izmerov, 1971). In addition, certain effects on the central nervous system can be studied by implanting electrodes in the brain, by electroencephalography, and by observing sleep patterns.

Congenital Malformations

During the last decade, animals have been used in testing drugs for teratogenicity, but comparative studies in spontaneously occurring malformations have been rather neglected. Birth defects are assuming increasing importance in human medicine, for the reasons mentioned in the first chapter.

Rather surprisingly, the cause of most human malformations is still unknown. Only a small proportion can be attributed to known genetic factors, recognized virus infections, or teratogenetic drugs. Increasingly sophisticated research is revealing that many of the defects are not hereditary, as had been supposed, but are due to environmental factors yet to be identified. Investigation of the causes of congenital abnormalities in man present special difficulties, one being that the fetus, unlike the child or adult, is not seen while the pathological processes are active.

In some respects, knowledge of spontaneous birth defects is more advanced with animals than with man. It is not uncommon for epidemics of congenital malformations to occur in domestic animals, where it is often a straightforward matter to trace the cause to infection, intoxication, deficiency, or genetic or environmental factors.

I shall indicate some of the conditions in animals which could be used as models for comparative studies. Let me first cite some examples involving infectious agents. Quite a number of viruses are known that may affect the fetus without killing it. In sheep, natural infection with bluetongue virus in pregnant ewes or vaccination with an attenuated strain may result in 20 percent of congenital encephalopathy and other defects in the lambs (Richards *et al.*, 1971); in cats, rats, and hamsters, certain parvoviruses produce cerebellar hypoplasia. There are several viruses that affect the fetus of pigs, calves, and sheep, leading sometimes to abortion or resorption of the fetus and sometimes to various types of congenital abnormality, especially of the nervous system (Done, 1968; Barlow *et al.*, 1970; Kahrs *et al.*, 1970). It is now recognized that there are some viruses which cause only subclinical infection in the adult animal, yet are pathogenic for the fetus and hence cause deformities. This points to a new line of investigation to pursue in human problems—to look for fetopathic effects from viruses that produce only silent infections in the mother.

Modern hygiene has led to many infections that used to occur early in life being deferred until later, when they may do more harm. In man, poliomyelitis and rubella are classic examples. We see the same thing happening in domestic animals; when young breeding females become infected during pregnancy, the fetus may be deformed.

Outbreaks of congenital abnormalities sometimes occur in farm animals due to ingestion of teratogenic substances. Ewes grazing pasture containing the plant *Veratrum californicum* in Idaho may give birth to lambs of which as many as 15 percent have brain and head deformities (Binns *et al.*, 1963). Lupins fed to pregnant cows can produce cleft palate, arthrogryposis, and other abnormalities in the fetus (Shupe *et al.*, 1967). An incident of considerable comparative interest occurred in Missouri recently (Menges *et al.*, 1970): 40 percent of the piglets in fourteen litters had congenital limb deformities. The cause was traced to the sows having eaten tobacco stalks in early pregnancy. There seems little doubt that the nicotine in the tobacco stalks was the offending substance. This finding gives greater significance to reports that below-average birth weights and increased neonatal mortality occur in babies from women who smoke, and it suggests further lines of inquiry.

In the nutrition field, deficiency of vitamin A is a not uncommon cause of abnormalities in calves. Deficiency of copper in ewes causes the nervous disease known as swayback in lambs. In this instance, there is not necessarily a deficiency of copper in the pasture; its absorption or utilization may be hindered by some other agent.

Genetics provides many examples of defects in domestic animals and in inbred lines of mice, while at the cytogenetic level there are many chromosome abnormalities known in animals that provide useful models for analogous human aberrations. Patterson (1968) and his colleagues at Philadelphia have studied a number of dogs with abnormalities of the heart and great vessels and have made comparisons with similar human defects. They are breeding the dogs to study the genetic and other factors involved in the hope of providing better understanding of the causes of these defects in man. Perhaps the most exciting research in comparative teratogenesis concerns the discovery of the effects of high environmental temperature on the fetus. A most illuminating incident occurred a few years ago in Sydney involving a number of malformations in a guinea pig colony (Edwards, 1969). Investigations revealed that the pregnant females had been exposed to high ambient temperature. Subsequent experimental work showed that exposure of pregnant guinea pigs or rats to high temperature resulted in a wide range of congenital malformations, including reduction in brain size and clubfoot. Presumably, fever due to an infection would have a similar effect. This work may well have important implications concerning congenital defects in man, including congenital idiocy. It is significant that more mental defectives are said to be born following early gestation in the summer.

Thus there are many spontaneously occurring conditions in animals which could be profitably exploited for comparative studies. All manner of causal factors can be analyzed in detail and the pathogenesis of defects studied during fetal development.

Reproduction and Population Control

From the practical point of view, reproduction has always been an important matter in farm livestock. Therefore, much scientific study has been devoted to the fundamental and applied aspects of the physiology of reproduction in farm and laboratory animals. In this field, the advantages of doing research with animals instead of man are even greater than with infectious disease: not only can we experiment freely, but reproduction in animals is not shrouded in taboos as certain aspects of it are in man—or were until very recently. Consequently, basic knowledge has been acquired which has made possible the development of technical methods which have been put into practice in animals on such matters as artificial insemination, long-term storage of semen, induction or inhibition of ovulation, *in vitro* fertilization, and transfer of ova and early embryos. Even more sophisticated manipulations are now being developed such as culturing embryos *in vitro,* sex determination, long-term storage of embryos, genetic engineering, and reproduction of exact copies of individuals— so-called cloning—by inserting the nuclei of somatic cells into ova (Edwards and Sharpe, 1971). In the brave new world of the near future, some or all of these techniques developed and put into practice with animals will be used in man.

The application of the knowledge of reproductive physiology gained from animals to the control of conception in man nowadays rightly receives a great deal of attention. The mechanisms whereby some animal communities control their population numbers have not yet been so much studied or exploited. It used to be thought that population numbers were limited only by food supply and disease, but it is now realized that social factors are also involved.

It is common knowledge that odors play a vital role in attracting male and female animals to each other at appropriate stages of their sexual cycle and in stimulating sexual activity. The odorous substances concerned are called pheromones. Pheromones are defined as volatile materials given off by one individual which affect the behavior and/or physiology of another individual in a highly specific way. They are analogous to hormones and are active in extremely small amounts. Only recently has serious attention been given to the possibility that they may play a part in human sexual physiology. Impetus was given to studying them in mammals by the discovery of Bruce and Parkes (1961) that when pregnant mice are exposed to the smell of a strange male, their fetuses die and are resorbed and the females come on heat. This phenomenon, known as the "Bruce effect," is being intensively studied to elucidate the mechanisms involved.

The next development in this field shows conclusively that pheromones play an active role in primates, although so far shown only among nonhuman primates. Michael and Keverne (1968) worked with rhesus monkeys in a fascinating series of experiments which showed that the male is stimulated sexually by pheromones from the vagina of sexually active females. They analyzed the active material which turned out to be a mixture of rather common chemical compounds. Further, they were able to prepare a mixture from pure chemicals which had the same effect on the male monkeys as did the natural secretions.

We are touching on a subject still surrounded by inhibitions in man and the next development brings us right into a delicate area. It has long been known that estrus cycles of some animals living in groups tend to be synchronized, for example, a group of young female pigs or mice often all come on heat at about the same time. It has also been reported that young women living together tend to have their menstrual cycles synchronized. Dr. Martha McClintock of Harvard (1971) recently investigated this phenomenon. The results led her to suggest that the influence of the girls on each other may be due to pheromones acting at a subliminal or subconscious level. If it can be confirmed that ovulatory cycles can be controlled in this way, it would open up remarkable possibilities for fertility control, and there may also be implications for psychology and psychiatry. It is said that Hippocrates attributed abortifacient powers to the sense of smell. Perhaps he was right. We do not yet know for certain whether human pheromones really do exist, but, if they do, there is already much basic knowledge about the effects, modes of action, and chemical composition of pheromones in animals to try out in man.

The role of pheromones in animal reproduction is but one example of a mechanism which can limit population growth when numbers become excessive and lead to crowding. It seems that most species studied, ranging from fishes to birds and mammals, have evolved social patterns of behavior linked with their physiology which have the effect of maintaining their numbers in ecological balance. In some species, the method involves possession of breeding territory by the male, with the females being sexually unresponsive to those males without territory. This remarkable system balances the reproductive rate with the living space available. In some other species, when overcrowding occurs, it is corrected by neglect of offspring by the parents, by lowered fertility, or by death from stress. Further study of animal behavior and reproductive physiology may reveal new mechanisms which may help industrialized man to avoid getting further out of balance with nature.

It must not be thought that these regulators of population size are as inevitable as the laws of physics and that something along these lines will come into play in time to save mankind from disastrous overpopulation. The regulators act only in the ecological environment in which the species has evolved; move a species to a new environment and often reproduction runs wild, as happened for example when European rabbits were taken to Australia. Similarly, farmers have learned how to raise domestic animals under intensive conditions where the natural checks are deliberately avoided. Civilized man has overcome the checks due to famine, disease, and predators, and has forgotten any social regulators there may have been in primitive human societies living in ecological balance with the surrounding fauna and flora. For the first time a species, man, has gained control over the environment and thus has become master of its own destiny, for better or for worse. Human society today is dependent on science, and only by further application of science can we hope to deal effectively with the population problem.

Conclusion

In conclusion I would like to emphasize that I have chosen these research anecdotes not so much for their intrinsic interest as to show the way that animal models can be used to advance medical science. In studying the history of discoveries, what matters is not *who* made *what* discovery, or *when* or *where* it was made, because none of this will occur again and there is no lesson to be learned from it. What does matter is *how* the discovery was made, because this will be repeated again and again. The more we understand about how past discoveries have been made, the better we are able to plan for future discoveries.

CHAPTER 3

COMPARATIVE STUDY OF INFLUENZA

Influenza provides a splendid illustration of the unity of medicine on two grounds: the exchange of knowledge of the disease as it affects both man and animals and the exchange of infection between man and animals.

That is my justification for making it the subject of this chapter, but I must admit that there is also another more personal reason. I am one of those who have been fascinated by the story that has unfolded over the last half century. The growth of our knowledge in this field constitutes one of the most exciting stories in the history of medicine and there are still many intriguing mysteries to puzzle over. A group of specialists called together by the World Health Organization stated: "Influenza is one of the most important infectious diseases still unconquered." That was in 1952, but the statement is still true today. We are, of course, talking about "true" influenza which occurs mostly in epidemics, and not about sporadic respiratory infections that are often loosely referred to as influenza.

Comparative Study of Influenza

Epidemiological Behavior

Epidemics recognizable from their description as probably
influenza have been recorded since before the birth of Christ.
During the 225 years from 1675 to 1900, twenty-two epidemics were described in sufficient detail for us to be reasonably
sure that they were influenza. That averages out at about one
every decade, but actually the intervals were very irregular.
The particular characteristics that lead one to identify an
epidemic as influenza are the clinical symptoms, especially the
sudden onset, a high attack rate but relatively low mortality,
short incubation period, and rapid spread of the disease in the
country followed by its disappearance.

It was only comparatively recently that the contagious nature of the disease was generally accepted. There is a good description of an epidemic in Philadelphia in 1793 by Robert
Johnson (1806). He postulated that the disease was propagated
at least to some extent by contagion, but the editor of Johnson's publication added a footnote saying that he disagreed,
as he believed the disease to be "*exclusively*" of atmospheric
origin . . . probably a deleterious gas." As recently as 1894
the eminent British epidemiologist Charles Creighton did not
believe influenza was spread by contagion. Even in those days
when few traveled faster than a horse could carry them, influenza spread so rapidly that people found it hard to believe it
did not travel on the wind. Recent discoveries about the way
virus diseases of animals spread from farm to farm suggest influenza may in fact spread on the wind.

Now let us look more closely at the influenza calendar, as
we may call it, over the last hundred years or so. There was
an unusual period of thirty-four years from 1855 to 1889 during which no epidemics were reported. Then came a serious
worldwide pandemic in 1889 and recrudescences during the

next four years. At the time, that visitation was referred to as Asiatic influenza because it came from eastern Russia. During the twenty-eight years after 1890, lesser epidemics occurred every two or three years, and then the greatest of all epidemics swept around the world in 1918.

The great pandemic of 1918–19 was called Spanish influenza, but there was really no justification for that name. It started as the First World War was ending, a time when there were movements of masses of people, many of them ill-nourished, poorly clothed, and living under crowded conditions. Influenza encircled the globe, killing an estimated 15 to 20 million people in twelve months, many more than were killed in the First World War during four and a half years. Never before or since has mankind suffered such a calamity. For the first time, influenza was associated with high mortality; moreover, it was people in the prime of life who were hardest hit.

Another curious feature that was out of character, one which still cannot be explained, was that there were three waves separated by only a few months. In some places those people who had been affected in the first or second wave resisted the infection in subsequent waves, but in other places an attack during one wave gave no protection in the next. Not only did these waves spread with disconcerting swiftness but the disease struck people suddenly, and many died within a few days of becoming ill. I am old enough to remember fellow schoolboys collapsing suddenly without any warning. A proportion of the patients developed heliotrope coloring of the lips and face. These patients often did not feel particularly ill and were even cheerful, but the doctors soon learned that heliotrope cyanosis usually meant death in less than forty-eight hours. The epidemic spread to outlying farming communities, and the only groups of human beings to escape were those on a few remote islands.

Eventually the pandemic burned itself out, and the disease returned to its normal behavior, that is, causing epidemics of a widespread nature every few years but without high mortality. There were epidemics in 1929, 1932, and 1937. During the Second World War, some of us were worried that there might be another pandemic like the one in 1918–19. Again there were mass movements of people, many of them in great misery, conditions which some thought may have been responsible for setting off the earlier pandemic. But to everyone's surprise, influenza was less prevalent than usual during the last world war and the immediate postwar years. One must conclude that mass misery does not itself lead to influenza pandemics, though it might explain the severity of the 1918–19 pandemic once the new strain had been generated. It was not until 1949 that an epidemic of any consequence occurred. That year it caused 2,200 deaths in Holland alone. In 1951 there was another rather severe epidemic which at its peak caused over 1,000 deaths a week in Britain.

Then, in 1957, the so-called Asian influenza spread swiftly around the world causing many illnesses and a moderate number of deaths. This was a much-publicized epidemic and at its peak caused 1,600 deaths a week in England and Wales. Actually this figure was lower than the mortality in 1932–33, which reached 2,000 a week. There were lesser epidemics every two or three years, and then in 1968 came the so-called Hong Kong flu which again spread rapidly around the globe. It caused considerable mortality in the United States in 1968–69, the figures reaching about the same as in 1957, but strangely it caused hardly any mortality in Europe although the infection was widespread. In the following winter it flared up again in Europe and this time was accompanied by considerable mortality, comparable with that in the United States in the previous year.

The following figures give an idea of the importance of an influenza epidemic. At the peak of the Hong Kong flu epidemic, about 1,700 were dying from it each week in 122 large cities in the United States. The total mortality from the epidemic has been estimated at between 20,000 and 80,000 for the United States. About 20 percent of the population became clinically ill, causing a loss of 35 million working days. The total economic loss was estimated at 4,600 million dollars.

That is a brief history of this remarkable and unique disease. After absences of up to thirty-four years, it suddenly reappears and rapidly spreads from country to country like a new disease, affecting a large proportion of people. Each major epidemic behaves as a truly new disease because there is no immunity from previous outbreaks and consequently people of all ages are affected. This conduct is quite unlike that of any other disease. Diseases such as measles and mumps confer lifelong immunity and therefore outbreaks are largely confined to children.

By now we have learned a great deal about influenza and the virus which causes it, but some mysteries still remain. In the following section I shall describe in greater detail how the picture has unfolded over the last fifty years or so.

The Influenza Virus

During the 1918–19 epidemic, numerous attempts were made to demonstrate a virus by filtering material from the throats and lungs of active and fatal cases and spraying it into the noses of volunteers. No transmission was achieved. In other experiments, attempts were made to transmit the disease by exposing volunteers to coughs and sneezes of affected persons. Again, the results were almost uniformly negative. Attempts to incriminate bacteria were equally unsuccessful. The effect of these experiments was merely to deepen the mystery surrounding the cause of influenza, and during the 1920s ignorance on the subject was admitted to be complete. In 1929 an authoritative textbook reviewing the difficulties of demonstrating a causal virus concluded: "There is little hope that they [the difficulties] will ever be overcome in the case of influenza" (Scott, 1929).

But in fact work that was to lead to the solution of the problem was already in progress before 1929, though in a quite unexpected quarter. I am, of course, referring to the work on influenza in swine originating in the Midwest. In 1919 the veterinarian Dr. J. S. Koen of Fort Dodge, Iowa, described the close similarity between a disease he regarded as influenza in swine and that in man. In view of the historic importance of Koen's observations, it is worth quoting his report: "Last fall and winter we were confronted with a new condition, if not a new disease. I believe I have as much to support this diagnosis in pigs as the physicians have to support a similar diagnosis in man. The similarity of the epidemic among people and the epidemic among pigs was so close, the reports so frequent, that an outbreak in the family would be followed immediately by an outbreak among the hogs, and vice versa, as to present a most striking coincidence if not suggesting a close relation between the two conditions. It looked like 'flu,' and until proved it was not 'flu,' I shall stand by that diagnosis" (Koen, 1919).

Influenza temporarily disappeared from the human community but recurred each autumn in swine. In 1928 Dr. C. N. McBryde and his coworkers successfully transmitted the disease from pig to pig by intranasal inoculation of mucus from the respiratory tract of sick pigs, but they failed to produce the disease with filtered material. The quest was then taken up by Richard Shope, who succeeded in transmitting the disease from pig to pig with filtrates (Shope, 1931). This may be said to be the discovery of the influenza virus, although like many discoveries it was not one sudden breakthrough but rather a series of findings. Shope's success encouraged the British workers Christopher Andrewes and Wilson Smith to re-investigate human influenza, which was again prevalent in England in 1933. A colony of ferrets became ill with a disease which was thought to be influenza, and this led Wilson Smith to try inoculation of this species with material from the throat of Christopher Andrewes, who had himself come down with influenza. The ferret proved to be just the experimental animal they long had sought, and soon they were able to show that human influenza was caused by a virus very similar to that causing swine influenza. Only later was it found that the disease in the colony of ferrets that had given this lead was not influenza but distemper (Andrewes, 1951).

When Shope tried inoculating ferrets intranasally, they struggled so much that he decided to anesthetize them. He found that when ferrets were inoculated under an anesthetic the influenza virus produced pneumonia. This finding in turn gave Andrewes and Smith the idea of inoculating mice intranasally under an anesthetic. The mice also developed pneumonia, and this provided a much better experimental animal than the ferret and opened the way for more extensive studies. A few years later Wilson Smith and Macfarlane Burnet developed methods of growing the virus in chick embryos. The virus was designated influenza type A to distinguish it from two other viruses which were isolated later and named types B and C. These latter are immunologically very different and are much less important, so I shall discuss only influenza type A.

During the 1940s and 1950s knowledge of the anatomy,

chemical composition, reproduction, and antigenic characters of the virus grew as virological techniques became more sophisticated. It would not be appropriate to describe this work here, but in order to explain the biological behavior of the virus it is necessary to mention its remarkable capacity to assume different antigenic disguises. Two types of change occur: gradual minor variations within the same subtype and sudden major changes to new subtypes.

Every year or so, minor variations occur in the antigenic makeup of the prevailing subtype. After two or three years, the changes are sufficient to enable the new variant to infect some people who had become immune to the previous strain and so cause a fresh epidemic, though usually not a very serious one, since many people have some immunity. Apart from this variation within a subtype, which is called antigenic drift, a new subtype appears every ten years or so. Most of the antigens of the new subtype are quite different from those of the previous one, so people have practically no immunity to it and a worldwide pandemic occurs like those of 1957 and 1968. This change is termed antigenic shift.

A strange feature of influenza epidemiology is that at any one time there exists in the world only one subtype and only one variant of it. Whenever a new variant or subtype appears, it ousts the previous one and, as far as we know, leads to its complete disappearance from the world. The reason is that infection with the new strain makes people strongly immune to the old strain, but old strains do not produce effective immunity to new strains. In other words the offspring confers protection against the parent and thus eliminates it, but the parent confers little or no protection against the offspring. It is as though each generation of children kill their parents and take over until they in turn are driven out by their own children. We know of no other virus that behaves in this way, and

71

it explains some features of the unique epidemic behavior of influenza.

Clearly it is of the greatest importance for us to understand more about how these changes in the antigens of influenza virus arise. The gradual antigenic drift producing small but significant variations is believed to be due to genetic mutations, and perhaps recombinations, plus selective survival, such as we are familiar with in more complicated organisms. These changes can be reproduced in the laboratory, at least to some extent, and there is no particular mystery about them. But antigenic shift—the sudden appearance of new subtypes that give rise to pandemics—is difficult to explain on this basis. The origin of new subtypes is the paramount problem of influenza and one about which speculation is rife. I believe we are now approaching the answer, but before I discuss that I must describe another aspect of influenza research, namely, influenza in animals.

Influenza in Horses

The history of human influenza epidemics abounds with reports that horses and various other species of animals were affected with a clinically similar disease about the same time as the people. The association of illness in animals with influenza in man has been so strong that some epidemiologists even used it as evidence that an epidemic which occurred during the siege of Troy was probably influenza "because it began upon the horses and dogs as so many historic influenzas have done" (Creighton, 1894). The epidemiologist C. A. Gill said in 1928 that there was a traditional belief that horses are invariably attacked during influenza epidemics.

Epidemics of an influenza-like illness in horses are reported to have been associated with human epidemics in 1688, 1727,

Comparative Study of Influenza

1733, 1737, 1750, 1760, 1771, 1788, 1837, and 1890 (Creighton, 1894). It was often said that the horses were affected a month or so before the people. One must of course regard these reports with considerable reserve because, whenever epidemics of any sort occurred, there was a tendency to associate them with illness in animals, and there was little understanding about the specificity of infectious diseases until about the middle of the last century.

But in 1956 Swedish workers reported serological evidence of influenza in horses, and shortly afterwards Sovinova, Tumova, and their colleagues in Prague isolated influenza type A virus from an epidemic of respiratory disease in horses (Sovinova *et al.*, 1958). Since then influenza has been found to cause epidemics in horses in many countries. Extensive epidemics occurred in the United States and Britain in 1963 and in Europe in 1965. The epidemic behavior and the clinical symptoms are remarkably similar to those in man.

We can now look back in history to the outbreaks described in horses and form an opinion on whether they were true influenza or one of the other diseases of horses we now recognize. There is little doubt that some of the horse outbreaks associated with human influenza were truly influenza. For example, in 1688 a contemporary observer said of the "horse cold" then prevalent: "It was generally observed, both in England and Ireland, that sometimes before the fever began [in the people], a slight but universal disease seized the horses" (Thompson, 1852). A very apt description of influenza outbreaks in horses we have seen in recent years would be a "horse cold" and a "slight but universal disease." I doubt if there is any other disease that would fit this description.

In 1728 and 1733 much the same story was recorded in Ireland: a widespread cough in the horses from which most recovered. Dr. Rutty (quoted by Creighton, 1894) reported: "In

1728 and 1733 it [the precedence of the horse cold] was most manifest, in which years a most severe cough seized almost all the horses, one or two months earlier than the men." In 1775 "catarrh" was prevalent among the horses in various parts of England and Wales. "This 'distemper' prevailed some time among horses before it attacked the human species. The cough harassed them severely and rendered them unfit for work, though few died" (Creighton, 1894).

We have a very full and graphic account of a serious epidemic of influenza of horses that swept right across North America in 1872 (Judson, 1874). It started near Toronto, and its progress across the continent was carefully recorded. As the disease continued to spread across the land, virtually all the horses were affected in each city within a few days after the arrival of the disease, paralyzing all transport in the area and disrupting business. That epidemic, unlike those referred to above, was not associated with an epidemic in man.

In 1889 an outbreak of disease started in horses before the human influenza epidemic. Thompson wrote a letter to the *British Medical Journal* early in December calling attention to the horse epidemic and predicting that there would be an epidemic in man (Thompson, 1890). However, the story is somewhat confused. The outbreak in horses started in September and reached epidemic proportions in October, November, and December in London. A clinical description given by Thompson (1890) suggests the horses may have been affected by "pink-eye" (infectious arteritis) and not true influenza. However, a detailed description given by Parsons (1891) suggests that arteritis and influenza may have both occurred in horses around that time. The human epidemic spread from eastern Russia and arrived in London in December. There were stories of disease thought to be influenza affecting horses and lambs about the same time. Parsons relates several instances where the circumstantial evidence suggested that people became infected from horses. Whether or not transmission between man and horses or sheep did really occur, there is little doubt that it was through human contacts that the influenza was transmitted to Britain from eastern Europe.

During the 1918–19 pandemic there were hardly any reports of influenza in horses, through Gill (1928) said horses were affected. In an article in the *Lancet* of March 1919 (Anonymous, 1919), there was a report of heavy mortality in wild baboons in South Africa attributed to the influenza and an outbreak in sheep in Westmorland thought to be influenza, but there is no mention of an outbreak of the disease in horses.

Indeed, so far in this century outbreaks of influenza in man on the one hand and in horses on the other do not seem to have coincided. A few isolated incidents occurred which suggested that some people had been infected from horses, but laboratory investigations showed that these were only coincidences. Two points should be borne in mind: firstly, the horse population has been greatly reduced since the 1920s; secondly, observers have adopted a more critical attitude and are conscious that the term "influenza" has been used loosely to describe various respiratory diseases of man and of animals. The stories of the association of influenza in man and horses in previous centuries were no longer taken seriously until the influenza virus was isolated from horses in 1956. Subsequent demonstration of an antibody against one of the equine subtypes in the sera of old people who had lived through the 1890 epidemic reopened the possibility that there may be a significant connection between influenza in man and in horses. I shall return to this point again after considering other animal hosts.

Influenza in Other Animals

On reading accounts of human influenza epidemics during the last several centuries, one comes across frequent mention of what was thought to be the same disease affecting many different species. Horses are most frequently mentioned, but this may have been partly due to the fact that they were so numerous and played such an important part in everyone's life before the motor car supplanted them. Probably dogs are mentioned next most commonly. This may have been partly because people are aware of the health of their pets. Various farm animals and wild animals are also mentioned. It is impossible to know what significance one should attach to these reports. No doubt many of them were mere coincidences, and the tendency in recent times has been to dismiss them as such. However, developments during the last decade or so indicate more attention should be paid to influenza in animals of all sorts. We now know that pigs became infected with the same virus as man in 1918–19 and again in 1969 (Kundin, 1970). Also we know that dogs and cats may be infected from contact with human cases (Nikitin *et al.*, 1972; Paniker and Nair, 1970), and that human strains will spread in certain species of nonhuman primates (Johnsen *et al.*, 1971). An epidemic in ferrets was reported due to the then-current human influenza strain (Bell and Dudgeon, 1948).

No one had seriously considered birds as hosts for influenza until Schäfer (1955) found that fowl plague virus belonged to this family of viruses. This highly lethal disease was first described nearly a hundred years ago, and its viral etiology was demonstrated as far back as 1900 by two Italian workers, Centanni and Savonuzzi. Influenza virus was isolated from ducks in 1956 by Koppel and his colleagues in Czechoslovakia (Koppel *et al.*, 1956) and Simmons in Britain (Simmons, 1956).

Comparative Study of Influenza

Since then influenza viruses have been found in many parts of the world causing disease in chickens, turkeys, quails, pheasants, terns, guinea fowls, and parrots. There is also serological evidence that influenza occurs in several species of wild birds, including some that migrate over long distances. Antibodies have been found in shearwaters caught off the Australian coast. These birds migrate as far north as the Aleutian Islands. The disease outbreaks in domestic poultry due to influenza viruses nearly all occur sporadically, which indicates that there is probably a reservoir in wild birds.

To sum up, we now know that the host range of the influenza virus includes man, pigs, horses, ferrets, dogs, cats, some nonhuman primates, and a large number of avian species. Mice, rats, hamsters, squirrels, mink, chipmunks (McQueen *et al.*, 1968), and even dolphins (Sigel *et al.*, 1971) also can be infected experimentally. We are obviously dealing with a parasite with a wide host range, and it is to be expected that it will be found in yet more species.

Relationship of Human and Animal Strains

Earlier I referred to the changes in antigenic makeup that take place in human strains of influenza virus. We must now consider the antigenic characters of the animal strains and their relationship to human strains. Let me first explain the antigenic structure of the virus.

The elementary bodies consist of a central nucleoprotein core and a lipoprotein envelope. There are three antigens, one in the nucleoprotein core and two in the envelope. The nucleoprotein antigen is exactly the same for all influenza type A viruses; this is the antigen by which one recognizes a virus as type A influenza and quite distinct from types B and

C. Since this antigen is identical in all human and animal strains, we need not discuss it further. This leaves the two envelope antigens, which are called hemagglutinin and neuraminidase. Both of these differ to a greater or lesser extent from one strain to another. Influenza type A strains have been divided into subtypes according to their hemagglutinin and neuraminidase antigens. Within a subtype there are some differences between strains with respect to these antigens, but between subtypes the differences are much greater and sometimes complete. Whether or not there is cross-immunity between strains depends on these antigens, so usually there is some degree of cross-immunity within a subtype but little or none between subtypes.

Now let us look at the range of human and animal strains in the light of their antigenic characters. There are three human subtypes, referred to as A0, A1, and A2; two horse subtypes referred to as Equi 1 and Equi 2; one swine subtype; and eight avian subtypes. Within most of the subtypes there are several strains which differ appreciably from each other but do overlap to some extent.

So far, eight different neuraminidase antigens have been identified, and four of these are shared between subtypes isolated from different species. The first is shared by human A0 and A1 and Swine, the second by human A2 and Avian 6, the third by Equi 1 and Avian 1 and 2, and the fourth by Equi 2 and Avian 7. The remaining four neuraminidase antigens are specific for Avian 3, 4, 5, and 8 and have not yet been found in subtypes from other species (Schild and Tumova, 1972).

Hemagglutinin antigens vary independently from the neuraminidase. They are also shared between subtypes, though not to the extent that was thought until quite recently. Several papers have been published describing an elaborate pattern of cross-reactions determined by serological tests which indicated that the hemagglutinin of every subtype was related directly or indirectly to that of every other. But recently it has been realized that the conventional serological tests are influenced by other viral components besides the hemagglutinin. When the tests are done with monospecific sera to purified hemagglutinin, fewer cross-reactions are found. The true interrelations according to these more critical tests have not yet all been worked out, but it has been shown that there is a definite crossing between A2 Hong Kong, Equi 2, and classical swine, and there are many crosses between the avian subtypes (Schild and Tumova, 1972).

When one reflects that antigens are an expression of genetic makeup, it follows that all subtypes are related genetically and that they all belong to one family. This implies that some have descended from others and that there has been interbreeding and exchange of various characters.

It has been known for some years that strains of influenza can be made to cross-breed in the laboratory and produce stable hybrids with some characters from each parent. Recently Webster and his collaborators (1971) showed that hybridization can also occur in living animals. They inoculated pigs and turkeys with two strains simultaneously and found that a new hybrid strain was produced which inherited some characteristics from each of the parent strains. The new strain remained stable after passage through animals. Later they merely exposed turkeys to others which had been inoculated with different strains and a hybrid strain was produced in the exposed turkeys.

So far, I have referred only to variation in the antigenic characters, but strains also differ in a number of other ways, the most important being host affinity. No difficulty was experienced in cross-breeding strains with different host affinities and belonging to different antigenic subtypes. New hybrids were produced with the host affinity of one parent combined with the antigenic character of the other parent. In the light of this work it is hard to escape the conclusion that the complex network of interrelationships of human and animal strains has been produced by hybridization occurring naturally.

The Origin of Pandemics

With most epidemic diseases, we know enough about the reservoirs of the infectious agent, the level of immunity in the population, and the means of transmission to be able to predict, within certain limits, the likelihood of an epidemic arising in the near future. This applies to influenza only so far as the prevailing subtype is concerned. We are completely in the dark about fresh pandemics, which so far have always taken us by surprise.

Earlier I referred to the origin of new subtypes that cause pandemics as the paramount problem of influenza research. The ultimate solution to the influenza problem would be to stop pandemics from arising, and I venture to suggest that this goal should not be regarded as beyond our reach. If we could discover the factors that lead to the emergence of new subtypes, we might be able to do something toward preventing a new one from arising. Or if we cannot stop it, perhaps we could learn where and when it is likely to appear and what will be its probable antigenic composition. That knowledge would enable vaccines to be prepared in advance and applied in such a way that the pandemic would be aborted. This is, of course, speculative and looking a long way ahead, but I believe it is now time that we start to give serious consideration to these possibilities.

One can think of four hypotheses to explain the origin of

new human subtypes: (1) a major mutation from a previous human subtype; (2) an animal strain with pre-existing potential human affinity suddenly finding its way into man; (3) adaptation of an animal strain to man, and (4) hybridization of a human and animal strain.

A major mutation of a human strain has probably been the most widely held hypothesis, at least until recently, but there are difficulties in accepting it. If it were possible for the virus to undergo such large mutations, the most likely time for them to occur would be when the greatest number of virus particles are being produced, that is, during pandemics or when they are waning. That possibly occurred during the unique pandemic of 1918–19, but during other pandemics the virus has remained constant. The major mutation hypothesis has, I think, become almost untenable in light of recent critical studies by Webster and Laver (1971, 1972) on the serology and biochemistry of the hemagglutinin antigens. They found that the hemagglutinin of an early example of the Hong Kong pandemic strain is completely different from that of the human strain which prevailed just previously. It seems improbable that such a complete serological and chemical change could take place by mutation; on the other hand, we know that antigens very similar to, if not identical with, those of the Hong Kong strain do exist in animal strains.

This leaves the three possibilities in which animal strains are implicated. Before considering these separately, I would like to present some background evidence which supports the idea that animal strains are involved in one way or another.

Pertinent information has been obtained from looking for antibodies in the sera of people of different ages. This was first done in an attempt retrospectively to connect the 1918–19 pandemic with swine influenza, and it is generally agreed that the swine subtype is a descendant of the virus that caused the great pandemic. Going back still further, it has been found that old people who were born before the 1890 pandemic have antibodies against the Equi 2 subtype and the human A2 subtype (Masurel, 1969). It may be significant that horses were said to be affected during that pandemic. It has already been mentioned that the 1957 pandemic strain is closely related to several avian strains, and the 1968 Hong Kong strain is closely related to Equi 2.

I believe that the body of evidence is now strongly in favor of the view that animal strains play a part in the genesis of new human pandemics, and it remains for us to consider how it comes about.

The second of the four hypotheses is that an animal strain with pre-existing potential human affinity suddenly finds its way into man. In this connection it should be mentioned that none of the presently known animal strains readily infect people who come into contact with infected animals. The only possible exceptions are that the swine subtype may sometimes infect people, and one of the horse subtypes infects people who are deliberately inoculated with it. However, there is no doubt that some influenza strains can cross the species barrier in the opposite direction, that is, from man to animal. Infection was readily transmitted to pigs in 1918–19 and in 1968, and occasional transmission to ferrets, dogs, and cats has taken place. This hypothesis of simple transfer from an animal reservoir does not fit with the fact that pandemics arise only infrequently. If potentially human strains existed in animals, one would expect transfer to occur frequently—in other words, for pandemics to arise frequently. One can only entertain this hypothesis if one assumes there are a number of potential human strains endemic in some animals that seldom come in contact with man. This is conceivable but farfetched, and I prefer alternative hypotheses.

Comparative Study of Influenza

We are seeking an explanation for a rare event, one that happens about once in ten years in the whole world. The explanation should take into account the serological links that we know exist between animal and human strains. Both the remaining hypotheses meet these theoretical requirements. They are adaptations of an animal strain to man and hybridization between a human and an animal strain.

Like many other viruses, influenza can be adapted to new hosts in the laboratory by inoculation with large doses and transfer from animal to animal. Under natural conditions the 1918–19 strain became adapted to pigs and, in doing so, largely lost its affinity for man; the Hong Kong strain isolated from pigs in Taiwan seems to be going the same way. The fact that the Hong Kong strain so very readily infects pigs suggests that it may have been originally a pig strain which crossed the species barrier into man and adapted to man so well that it was able to cause a pandemic.

The mechanism of adaptation with all viruses is assumed to be mutation with selective survival. It is worth listing the factors that may be involved in a virus adapting to a new host and seeing how they may be involved in the problem we are considering.

1. *Age susceptibility.* The very young are usually much more susceptible to infection than older individuals; thus, exposure of babies to infected animals could be a factor.

2. *Dose of virus.* Massive doses are more likely to initiate infection. This could occur when an individual enters a confined space housing many infected animals.

3. *Passage.* Crowding would provide favorable conditions for transfer to a second and third individual.

4. *Statistical probability.* Exposure to a large number of people would increase the likelihood of the virus meeting an occasional individual who is exceptionally susceptible.

5. *Host genetics.* Some races or genetic groups may be more susceptible than others to the animal strain.

6. *Decreased host resistance.* Decreased resistance may be due to stress, malnutrition, exposure to cold, or other infections.

This leads us to the fourth and last hypothesis, namely hybridization, which, as already mentioned, occurs readily when two strains of influenza are present simultaneously in the same host. For a new human subtype to arise in this way, a dual infection of man with a human strain and an animal strain would be required. We know that most strains are not strictly specific for only one host. In any case, the animal strain need not be capable of setting up a clinically obvious infection in man; it would be sufficient if it were able to undergo just one abortive cycle in the cells of the respiratory tract. In the reshuffle of genes, new hands would be dealt, some of which would contain the hemagglutinin from the animal strain combined with the host affinity of the human strain. Such an event is theoretically quite possible and might be expected to occur occasionally and be favored by the same six factors listed a moment ago as favoring adaptation of an animal strain to man. In light of our present knowledge, this seems to be the most likely way that new human subtypes are created.

Let us now look at another aspect of the origin of pandemics, namely, the geographic region where they start. It is quite remarkable that most pandemics are reported to have started somewhere about the center of the Eurasian landmass. Gill (1928) states that "all authorities are agreed that pandemics of influenza can almost invariably be traced to 'the silent spaces' of Asia, Siberia, and Western China." Creighton wrote in 1894: "In the early winter of 1889 the newspapers began to publish long telegrams on the influenza in Moscow, St. Petersburg, Berlin, Paris, Madrid, and other foreign capi-

tals. This epidemic wave, like those immediately preceding it
. . . in 1833, 1837 and 1847, and like one or more, but by no
means all, of the earlier influenzas, had an obvious course
from Asiatic and European Russia towards Western Europe.
. . . The Russian Army Medical Report favoured the view
that the birthplace of this pandemic in the autumn of 1889
was an extensive region occupied by nomadic tribes in the
northern part of the Kirghiz Steppe. There is evidence of its
rapid progress westwards over Tobolsk to the borders of
European Russia."

The great 1918-19 pandemic started with a rather mild
form of the disease in the spring of 1918, while the First
World War was still being fought and there was revolution in
Russia. This mild spring wave was reported in Europe and
in China and Japan, but there is no definite record of where
it started. However, Gill (1928) states that the site of origin
"has again been traced with some certainty to Central Asia."

The next two pandemics, those of 1957 and 1968, first became known to the world when they caused outbreaks in
southern China. Unfortunately, for political reasons it has so
far not been possible to find out if they arose there or came
from the interior, but quite likely the Chinese authorities
have valuable information on this point.

The region implicated by these reports is a vast, ill-defined
area. Some three thousand miles and enormous mountain
ranges separate the eastern boundary of European Russia
from southern China. Nevertheless, there must be something
of special significance in so many pandemics starting in the
same part of the world. It might be because there is so much
intimate human-animal contact there. In Mongolia and in
parts of eastern European Russia there are vast numbers of
domestic animals, the birdlife is said to be almost unimagin-
ably rich, and wild animals are plentiful. In many of these

areas newborn animals are tended in the same yurts where the people live with their babies. In parts of China it is also common for animals and people to occupy not only the same house but the same room. This close association between man and animals has been going on in central Asia for seven thousand years.

If we look again at the list of factors that favor a virus crossing the species barrier, we see that several of the factors might well occur more frequently in that part of the world than elsewhere. For example, where animals share a dwelling with people, newborn babies could be exposed to an animal influenza.

Parasites flourish when their hosts become numerous and crowded. The human race has become very numerous and crowded. Modern transport and large aggregations of people have provided ideal conditions for the spread of this airborne parasite. Influenza pandemics could well become increasingly serious, and there is no reason why there should not be another catastrophic one like that of 1918–19 or even worse. One of the avian strains causes practically 100 percent mortality in chickens. Present methods of vaccination and chemoprophylaxis are unlikely to do more than protect a few selected people, and quarantine measures are quite ineffective. Influenza is a disease unlike any other: it causes global pandemics which we cannot yet control. Therefore we should not confine our approach to measures appropriate to other diseases. I feel that what is needed now is an attempt at a more radical solution—to make a concerted attack on the paramount problem of the origin of pandemics.

There is mounting evidence that animal strains are involved, and we have a good indication of the part of the world where the pandemic is most likely to arise. I suggest there should be a study of the ecology of man and animals throughout Gill's "silent spaces," and selected species should be sampled for antibodies against influenza. A network of sentinel posts should be set up at strategic points to maintain a constant surveillance, watching antibody levels in animals and man and isolating strains whenever outbreaks occur. Obviously, international collaboration would be essential. But surely in this space age countries of all political ideologies can combine in a modest crusade against the common enemy of all mankind. Pandemic influenza is a global disease. This, then, is the story so far, and clearly there are exciting installments yet to be written. Apart from the paramount problem of the origin of new pandemic strains, we are still quite ignorant about the mechanisms that determine host affinity and virulence, and we can only partly explain why, during an epidemic, some people escape while their neighbors fall ill. And I have no doubt that some unexpected turns lie ahead because flu has a well-earned reputation for surprises. Both workers and watchers must have often experienced the feeling voiced by Keats:

> *Then felt I like some watcher of the skies*
> *When a new planet swims into his ken,*
> *Or like stout Cortez when with wond'ring eyes*
> *He star'd at the Pacific, and all his men*
> *Look'd at each other with a wild surmise—*
> *Silent upon a peak in Darien.*

About the Author

ABOUT THE AUTHOR

An international authority on comparative medicine and a consultant in that field to the World Health Organization in Geneva, W. I. B. Beveridge is a professor of animal pathology in the University of Cambridge School of Veterinary Medicine.

Dr. Beveridge was born in Junee, Australia. He attended the University of Sydney where he earned the degrees of Bachelor of Veterinary Science in 1930 and Doctor of Veterinary Science in 1941. He received the Master of Arts degree from Cambridge in 1947 and was awarded the honorary degree of Doctor of Veterinary Medicine by Hannover Veterinary University in Germany in 1963.

Before joining the Cambridge faculty in 1947, Dr. Beveridge served as a research bacteriologist at McMaster Animal Health Laboratory, Sydney; as a Commonwealth Fund service fellow at Rockefeller Institute, Princeton, New Jersey, and at the Bureau of Animal Industry in Washington, D.C.; as a research officer in virology at Walter and Eliza Hall Institute for Medical Research in Melbourne; and as a visiting worker at the Pasteur Institute in Paris.

Dr. Beveridge is the author of *The Art of Scientific Investigation*. His publications include numerous articles on infectious diseases of man and domestic animals. He also has written extensively on epidemiology, veterinary public health, and comparative medicine.

References

REFERENCES

Andrewes, C. H. (1951). Influenza virus and the beginning of its study in the laboratory. *Med. Press*, 225, No. 5844.

Anonymous (1919). Does epidemic influenza affect the lower animals? *Lancet*, March 29, 1919, 520. Annotation.

Barlow, R. M., A. C. Gardiner, I. Janice Storey, and J. S. Slater (1970). Experiments in Border disease. II. Some aspects of the disease in the foetus. *J. Comp. Path.*, 80:635–643.

Bell, F. R., and J. A. Dudgeon (1948). An epizootic of influenza in a ferret colony. *J. Comp. Path.*, 58:167–171.

Binns, W., L. F. James, J. L. Shupe, and G. Everett (1963). A congenital cyclopian-type malformation in lambs induced by maternal ingestion of a range plant *Veratrum californicum*. *Am. J. Vet. Res.*, 24:1164–1175.

Bittner, J. J. (1936). Some possible effects of nursing on the mammary gland tumor incidence in mice. *Science*, 84:162.

Bruce, H. M., and A. S. Parkes (1961). An olfactory block to implantation in mice. *J. Reprod. Fert.*, 2:195–196.

Bulletin of the World Health Organization (1972). *Virus-associated immunopathology: animal models and implications for human disease*. In press.

Centanni and Savonuzzi (1900). Cited by E. L. Stubbs in *Diseases of poultry*, edited by H. E. Biester and L. H. Schwarte. 4th ed. 1959. Iowa State University Press.

Charney, J., and D. H. Moore (1971). Neutralization of murine mammary tumour virus by sera of women with breast cancer. *Nature*, London, 229:627–628.

Chopra, H. C., and M. M. Mason (1970). A new virus in a spontaneous tumour of a rhesus monkey. *Cancer Res.*, 30:2081–2086.

Churchill, A. E., and P. M. Biggs (1968). Herpes-type virus isolated in cell culture from tumours of chickens with Marek's disease. II. Studies *in vivo*. *J. Nat. Cancer Inst.*, 41:951–956.

Cornelius, C. E. (1969). Animal models—a neglected medical resource. *New Engl. J. Med.*, 281:934–944.

Creighton, C. (1894). *A history of epidemics in Britain*, vol. 2. 2nd ed. 1965. Frank Cass & Co. Ltd., London.

Done, J. T. (1968). Congenital nervous diseases of pigs: a review. *Lab. Anim.*, 2:207–217.

Edwards, M. J. (1969). Congenital defects in guinea-pigs. Fetal resorptions, abortions and malformations following induced hyperthermia during early gestation. *Teratology*, 2:313–328.

Edwards, R. G., and D. J. Sharpe (1971). Social values and research in human embryology. *Nature*, London, 231:87–91.

Eidson, C. S., S. H. Kleven, and D. P. Anderson (1972). Vaccination against Marek's disease. In *Oncogenesis and Herpesviruses*, edited by P. M. Biggs, G. B. de Thé, and L. N. Payne. IRAC Scientific Publication No. 2. International Agency for Research on Cancer, Lyon.

Gill, C. A. (1928). *The genesis of epidemics*. Baillière, Tindall & Cox Ltd., London.

Helder, A. W., F. J. Blomjous, T. M. Feltkamp-Vroom, and J. J. van Loghem (1971). Microtubules of systemic lupus erythematosus. *Lancet*, June 5, 1971, 1183.

Izmerov, N. F. (1971). Some biological aspects of air pollution. WHO *Chronicle*, 25:51–57.

Jarrett, W. F. H. (1972). Feline leukaemia. In *International review of experimental pathology*, edited by G. W. Richter and M. A. Epstein, pp. 244–263. Academic Press.

Johnsen, D. O., W. L. Wooding, Prayot Tanticharoenyos, and Chalobon Karnjanaprakorn (1971). An epizootic of A2/Hong Kong/68 influenza in gibbons. *J. Infect. Dis.*, 123:365–370.

Johnson, R. (1806). *An inaugural dissertation on the influenza (University of Pennsylvania, 1793)*. Published by Thomas & William Bradford, Philadelphia.

Jones, T. C. (1969). Mammalian and avian models of disease in man. *Fed. Proc.*, 28:162–169.

Judson, A. B. (1874). Report on the origin and progress of the epizootic among horses in 1872, with a table of mortality in New York. *Veterinarian*, London, 47(N. S. 20):492–521.

Kahrs, R. F., F. W. Scott, and A. de Lahunta (1970). Epidemiological observations on bovine viral diarrhoea–mucosal disease, virus induced congenital cerebellar hypoplasia and ocular defects in calves. *Teratology*, 3:181–184.

Koen, J. S. (1919). A practical method for field diagnosis of swine diseases. *Am. J. Vet. Med.*, 14:468–470.

Koppel, Z., J. Vrtiak, M. Vasil, and S. Spiesz (1956). A mass infection of ducklings in East Slovakia characterized by signs of infectious sinusitis. *Veterinarstvi*, 6:267–268.

Kundin, W. D. (1970). Hong Kong A2 influenza virus infection among swine during a human epidemic in Taiwan. *Nature*, London, 228:857.

Leader, R. W., and Isabel Leader (1971). *Dictionary of comparative pathology and experimental biology*. W. B. Saunders Company, Philadelphia.

Lewis, R. M., and R. S. Schwartz (1971). Canine systemic lupus erythematosus. Genetic analysis of an established breeding colony. *J. Exp. Med.*, 134:417–438.

References

McBryde, C. N., W. B. Niles, and H. E. Moskey (1928). Investigations on the transmission and etiology of hog flu. *J. Am. Vet. Med. Ass.*, 26:331–346.

McClintock, Martha K. (1971). Menstrual synchrony and suppression. *Nature*, London, 229:244–245.

McQueen, J. L., J. H. Steele, and R. W. Robinson (1968). Influenza in animals. *Adv. Vet. Sci.*, 12:285–336.

Masurel, N. (1969). Relation between Hong Kong virus and former human A2 isolates and the A/Equi 2 virus in human sera collected before 1957. *Lancet*, May 3, 1969, 907–910.

Menges, R. W., L. A. Selby, C. J. Marienfeld, W. A. Aire, and D. L. Greer (1970). A tobacco-related epidemic of congenital limb deformities in swine. *Environ. Res.*, 3:285–302.

Michael, R. P., and E. B. Keverne (1968). Pheromones in the communication of sexual status in primates. *Nature*, London, *218*, 746–749.

Moore, D. H., J. Charney, B. Kramarsky, E. Y. Lasfargues, N. H. Sarkar, M. J. Brennan, J. H. Burrows, S. M. Sirsat, J. C. Paymaster, and A. B. Vaidya (1971). Search for a human breast cancer virus. *Nature*, London, 229:611–615.

Murray, J. A. (1911). *Cancerous ancestry and the incidence of cancer in mice*. 4th Scientific Report, Investigations of the Imperial Cancer Research Fund, pp. 114–130.

Nikitin, T., D. Cohen, J. D. Todd, and F. S. Lief (1972). *Hong Kong influenza in dogs*. Bull. World Health Organ. In press.

Paniker, C. J. K., and C. M. G. Nair (1970). *Infection of A2 Hong Kong influenza virus in domestic cats*. Bull. World Health Organ., 43:859–862.

Parsons, F. (1891). *Report to local government board on the influenza of 1889–90*. H. M. Stat. Off., London.

Patterson, D. F. (1968). Animal models of congenital heart disease, with special reference to patent ductus arteriosis in the dog. *Animal Models for Biomedical Research*. Nat. Acad. Sciences, Washington, Publication No. 1594, pp. 131–156.

Richards, W. P. C., G. L. Crenshaw, and R. B. Bushnell (1971). Hydranencephaly of calves associated with natural bluetongue virus infection. *Cornell Vet.*, 61:336–348.

Schachter, J., M. G. Barnes, J. P. Jones, Jr., E. P. Engelman, and K. F. Meyer (1966). Isolation of Bedsoniae from the joints of patients with Reiter's syndrome. *Proc. Soc. Exp. Biol. Med.*, 122:283–285.

Schäfer, W. (1955). Verglichende sero-immunologische Untersuchungen über die Viren der Influenza und der klassischen Geflügelpest. *Z. Naturf.*, 10b: 81–90.

Schild, G. C., and B. Tumova (1972). *Antigenic relationships between influenza A viruses of human, porcine, equine and avian origin*. Bull. World Health Organ. In press.

Schlom, J., S. Spiegelman, and D. Moore (1971). RNA-dependent DNA polymerase activity in virus-like particles isolated from human milk. *Nature*, London, 231:97–100.

Scott, W. M. (1929). The influenza group of bacteria: the aetiology of epidemic influenza. In *M. R. C. system of bacteriology in relation to medicine*, 2:326–394. H. M. Stat. Off., London.

Selby, L. A., C. J. Marienfeld, W. Heidlage, H. T. Wright, and V. E. Young (1971). Evaluation of a method to estimate the prevalence of congenital malformations in swine, using a mailed questionnaire. *Cornell Vet.*, 61: 203–213.

Shope, R. E. (1931). Swine influenza. III. Filtration experiments and etiology. *J. Exp. Med.*, 54:373–385.

Shupe, J. L., W. Binns, L. F. James, and R. F. Keeler (1967). Lupine, a cause of crooked calf disease. *J. Am. Vet. Med. Ass.*, 151:198–203.

Sigel, M. M., J. C. Lee, and W. G. Gilmartin (1971). *Virological studies in dolphins.* Conf., Internat. Ass. for Aquatic Animal Medicine, Guelph, Ontario (April, 1971).

Simmons, G. B. (1956). Cited by C. H. Andrewes and G. Worthington (1959). Bull. World Health Organ., 20:435–443.

Sovinova, O., B. Tumova, F. Pouska, and J. Nemec (1958). Isolation of a virus causing respiratory disease in horses. *Acta Virol.*, Prague, 2:52–61.

Thompson, E. Symes (1890). *Influenza or epidemic catarrhal fever. An historical survey of past epidemics in Great Britain from 1510 to 1890.* Percival & Co., London.

Thompson, T. (1852). *Annals of influenza or epidemic catarrhal fever in Great Britain from 1570 to 1837.* The Sydenham Society, London.

Webster, R. G., C. H. Campbell, and A. Granoff (1971). The "in vivo" production of "new" influenza A viruses. I. Genetic recombination between avian and mammalian influenza viruses. *Virology*, 44:317–328.

Webster, R. G., and W. G. Laver (1971). Antigenic variation in influenza virus; biology and chemistry. *Prog. Med. Virol.*, 13:271–338.

Webster, R. G., and W. G. Laver (1972). *The origin of pandemic influenza.* Bull. World Health Organ. In press.

Index

INDEX

Index

FROM FRONT FLAP

The author desc
studies in cancer,
neuropathology, i
tal defects, menta
population regula
of these subjects
reaching implica
medicine are be
section he asser
about the origin
demics. He poi
probably resul
man and anim
and that the us
appears to be
He emphasize
investigation
the hope of pr

W. I. B. Be
animal pathol
bridge, Engla
World Veterin
number of ye
parative med
Organization
Scientific Inv

FRONTIERS IN COMPARATIVE MEDICINE

by W. I. B. Beveridge

The Wesley W. Spink Lectures on Comparative Medicine, Volume 1

In this initial volume of the series to be based on the Wesley W. Spink Lectures on Comparative Medicine, Dr. Beveridge, the noted British scientist, discusses the contributions to human medicine resulting from studies of disease in animals. The book serves as an excellent introduction to this important aspect of science, suitable for general readers as well as for those studyin or working in the medical, biological, or social sciences.

Dr. Beveridge examines the methodology of comparative science and tells of the remarkable series of key discoveries of disease agents which have emerged from research on animals. He explains the reasons for the success of animal studies in connection with human disease and makes a strong case for more research on naturally occurring animal models.